Fix Gluten Sensitivity

and

Heal your Gut

Improve Overall Health & Multiple Issues

Second Edition

Matthew Stubbs

Preface

I am not a medical doctor; Therefore I cannot practice medicine and nothing in this educational book should be construed otherwise; Apparently according to the law, only medicines can treat diseases and only doctors can diagnose them; I do not make any attempt to diagnose, treat, or recommend treatment for any disease(s); Gluten sensitivity is not a disease, and the contents of this book deal with addressing this non-disease condition; I do not recommend any medicines in this book, nor do I suggest that you forego the use of any medicines prescribed by your doctor or make substitutions for medical treatments without consulting your doctor; Accordingly, the content of this book is for informational and educational purposes only, and nothing herein should be construed or interpreted as contrary to the statements in this paragraph; Since I have conducted no personal scientific research, testing, or studies, all statements or claims herein about the potentially harmful effects of glyphosate and genetically engineered foods have been made and asserted by other people/groups and are not my claims— as such I accept no liability for the validity, integrity, or methods behind any such claims, data, or statements; any other statements are only my personal opinion. I accept no responsibility or liability for how you or anyone might make use of the contents herein; if you have a serious medical condition or disease, you are advised to work with a medical doctor. You are also advised to consult with your doctor before taking any actions or taking any supplements related to the information herein so they can evaluate and advise you based upon your personal situation, condition, needs, etc.

Table of Contents

Chapter 1: Introduction

Allow me to start out simply and briefly. Later on, things will have to get a bit more complicated and lengthy in order for you to fully understand and fix your gluten intolerance as well as heal your gut. However, I will do my best to keep it simple and easy enough for you to comprehend and apply. I will also use metaphors, put things in layman's terms, and give summaries.

While this book is primarily oriented towards fixing gluten sensitivity or intolerance, it also has a ton of good information about healing the gut and also relates to improving your overall health. In other words, even if you don't have gluten intolerance you can still get a ton of benefit from this book and program.

You see, my journey began by figuring out how to fix my gluten sensitivity, but that led me to discover a more general and fundamental problem. So, this book reveals a couple of core issues; Understanding and addressing these issues will help you in many ways far beyond the gluten intolerance, which turns out to really just be a symptom.

Therefore, using the program and solution I came up with to fix gluten sensitivity will very probably help you heal or improve multiple health issues with which you may also be dealing. These may include type II diabetes, obesity, chronic fatigue, irritable bowel syndrome, leaky gut, Crohn's, ADHD, depression, Parkinson's, Alzheimer's, Dementia, insomnia, and many others. I don't mean to suggest or claim this book and program can cure diseases.

However, many things in that list aren't diseases; Furthermore, it is known that things can be done even for "incurable diseases" that can lessen their impacts, improve quality of life, and slow their progression. So, this book may help do some of that. Even if that is not the case, this 60-day program includes multiple practices that are fundamentally healthy, which means that your overall health will improve.

It is fairly common knowledge that many health issues begin and relate to impaired gut health and poor diet. What this book provides you is the specific and detailed information that you need to cleanse your gut, repair the damage, and restore multiple parts of its function. But even beyond that, this book shows you the likely culprit that caused your poor gut health in the first place so that you can eliminate the cause of the problem. In other words, you can both heal your gut and keep it healthy from this point forward.

In terms of the poor diet aspect, the dietary changes and supplements recommended go a step further in order to resolve the many consequences and side effects of poor gut health along with the likely culprit or core problem. All combined, this book will address the three primary areas; It will save you a lot of time, research, and trying to figure things out for yourself–or having to buy, read, and study multiple books. In short, this book provides the details you need to know as well as a comprehensive yet simple plan to enable you to fix your gut, stop doing what damages it, and make healthy changes to what you put in your body from now on.

By reading this book you will get the details, knowledge, and insights to understand exactly how the strategies and plan I suggest for dealing with gluten can actually work to resolve it–as well as improve multiple common health issues and conditions. In other words, this is a powerful and effective program to use for a wide variety of health issues and leads to improving your overall health. The detailed program is laid out in an easy to follow timetable that walks you through a series of steps; Just follow the simple steps 1, 2, 3… With that said, let's jump in and begin.

After eating bread and gluten foods for about forty-five years, I developed gluten intolerance–it is now more commonly being called "gluten sensitivity". So, I researched how to fix the issue, but there didn't appear to be any actual solutions available. Everything I read on the subject just advised me to stop eating gluten. This same thing has obviously happened to most people that have an issue with gluten because it is nearly a catch phrase these days to say, "I'm gluten free". A walk down a supermarket isle, or even a glance at many restaurant menus, reveals "Gluten Free" is all the rage and has become part of our modern vocabulary. In fact, if you spend just a half hour researching gluten sensitivity on the internet, you will find that nearly everything you read will say there is no solution except to avoid eating gluten.

But again, I ate it with no issue for my whole life, but now suddenly I have some problem with eating gluten and am supposed to believe that it has no real solution? This made no sense to me at all. Well, millions of people now have this apparently mysterious condition and many of them ask that very same question. Why is it that it seems to have appeared out of nowhere and affected so many people? What is going on here? What is causing this? In this book we will discover the very likely cause and use this knowledge to implement a real solution.

Is the whole "Gluten Free" thing just some fad or a marketing campaign? To those that don't have the problem/intolerance (yet), it may seem so; Actually, part of the product labeling is simply marketing, which will be explained later. But, for the people that suffer the symptoms and effects of gluten intolerance, I can assure you it is a real thing. It just happens to be that it isn't fully understood, or worse yet, that it is misunderstood.

So I didn't settle for the advice to simply stop eating gluten. I will explain in the next chapter why it is that I simply didn't accept it, nor accept the fate of how it would impact the rest of my life. I will also explain why I don't think you should settle for this non-solution either.

What I personally did was to delve into the issue and do a lot of research and study about it. I spent countless hours doing that. I got deeply into understanding what gluten is, how it is digested, where it comes from, and what it is about those food sources that is very likely the cause of the actual problem. After quite some time and effort, I think I discovered what is really going on. This then allowed me to come up with a pragmatic solution and strategy to deal with and fix it.

I then took action. I tested out my theory and implemented my strategy. I'm happy to report that I fixed my gluten sensitivity. I can eat gluten again! I can now enjoy the many foods that contain it, without any reactions, symptoms, or issues. I fixed my gluten sensitivity and you can too!

In this book I will basically walk you through my own journey in the order that I undertook it because it worked for me. So, re-tracing my steps lays out a sensible and logical overall approach and way to understand what is going on. There are some parts that are presented a bit out of order from my journey and discoveries to be more organized and make more sense.

Personally I think that to really fix any problem there are some requirements. I think you need to understand the problem and related components at a fairly deep level. This rather detailed understanding achieves multiple things: it gives your mind the information it needs to see how any proposed solution can even be possible and work; it gives you the will, persistence, and motivation to take the required actions.

Put another way, if I don't provide you with the somewhat full and detailed understandings, then you would be left with two alternatives: to reject it out of hand because you cannot see how my solution makes any sense, or might be contrary to what you have thus far been exposed to and believe; to take my solution on rather blind faith. In my opinion, the former dooms you to suffer gluten intolerance, or to be deprived of wonderful foods by simply avoiding gluten. The latter blind faith approach I think will deprive you of the confidence, will, motivation, and persistence you will need to fix the problem thru action over time.

The blind faith approach might also mean you don't implement the solution as well because you personally lack the knowledge and comprehension that led to it. So, I know we might go into what some readers might think are "too many technical details", but for the aforementioned reasons I think they are important and quite possibly required. This book is fairly short, so even if they aren't required there isn't much harm done. Besides which, you will have some more knowledge than you started with–and that is rarely a bad thing.

Here is an overview of the flow and contents of the book. I will begin with a bit of my own personal story. While it may seem rather trivial, it will bring out some very important points that I will tie into and draw upon later in the book. Next we will go a bit more into what I've just mentioned about why you can actually solve/fix your gluten intolerance and not just avoid gluten.

Next we will shift gears and cover the more technical stuff and Biochemistry of gluten and how it is digested. That is going to help reveal the actual problem and solution when we tie it into some other chapters' information–like the next chapter where we locate the likely cause/culprit. That technical info will also help you understand why my solution will work to actually fix your gluten intolerance.

The rest of the book then begins by putting the pieces together and seeing the overall solution. That solution to fix the problem is broken down into three easy to understand steps or parts. Some of these have multiple parts, and each of them are covered in detail in their own chapter. Just follow those steps and the plan 1, 2, 3, etc. and you can stop having to be gluten free and experience many other health improvements!

After that I will introduce a general understanding about how the body adapts to and handles different things, which relates to the solution/strategy (and also why total gluten avoidance actually may do more harm than good). We will then talk about some advice to ensure the problem stays fixed, and what to do if you experience a bit of relapse.

We will conclude by briefly discussing a holistic approach to health that will quite likely aid in your healing–because basically to fix your gluten intolerance you are actually healing something that is damaged but can be repaired and healed. Nobody mentioned that to you did they? Nope, they just told you to not eat gluten. Well, that's the majority's opinion; I think it was Mark Twain that said, "When you find yourself on the side of the majority…it's time to reconsider."

Taken together then, this book provides you what you need to know to fix your gluten intolerance and very likely multiple other issues you may have going on as well. You will then be able to go back to eating all the wonderful foods you love that have gluten in them. In

Chapter 2: My Personal Story

I'm fifty years old now and grew up in a family with seven children. I was lucky enough to have a mother that was a full-time homemaker. All of those things taken together meant that I was raised almost entirely on home cooked meals. We barely ate any processed foods. We had almost no soda, instant dinners, or fast food. In fact, we rarely ate out at restaurants due to the cost and large family issues such as seating and the noise we made. But on our birthdays we got to pick what we wanted for dinner, which sometimes was cooked at home, but sometimes it meant eating out. Even so, the type and quality of food in restaurants was much different back then, and no one picked their birthday dinner to be at a fast food joint.

As a child, and compared to my schoolmates, my siblings and I felt a bit deprived. Of course we had sack lunches and I remember being jealous of the kids that got school lunches. I even wanted school lunches so much that I volunteered to work in the kitchen, which earned me a free hot lunch. On sleepovers with friends I was delighted to get things like frozen pizza, sodas, junk foods, and pre-sweetened cereal for breakfast. Of course with maturity and hindsight I am now thankful for my mother's cooking and the healthy food I was raised on.

One of the things that all my siblings and I did love and appreciate at the time was my mom's homemade bread. She had learned to make it from her best friend's mother because she enjoyed it so much. It had many grains in it and was half & half white flour and wheat flour. It would take her hours to make that bread. But, she would make six loaves at a time and freeze three of them. She used an old KitchenAid mixer for the first part, but then all the rest was done by hand. I recall watching her make bread many times and go through about a half dozen different techniques of kneading it: knuckle kneading, making long slabs and slapping them, folding and kneading again, karate chops, etc. The smell of it baking is one of those things that gets imprinted on your memory for the rest of your life.

Everyone loved my mother Nan's bread, which included our friends. We had one friend of the family that would miraculously show up unannounced nearly every time she would make bread–which wasn't a set day. So we always joked at his amazing intuition or psychic fresh bread detection ability–it was simply uncanny. When people would comment about how good Nan's bread was and ask her secret, she would explain that was because it was made with love and she put love into it with her hands.

Now I/we ate that bread as toast for breakfast. I ate that bread daily in my lunch sandwiches. We ate it often at dinner with soup, spaghetti, and other meals. It went into meatloaf and stuffing, and was made into breadcrumbs for salads. Even after her children had moved out of the house she would continue to make it, and we'd get a loaf to take home when we would visit. So why do I tell this story? Well the bottom line is that I ate a hell of a lot of bread in my days and continued to eat bread for about forty-six years with no problem at all.

Then something happened. Something changed. I started having a variety of issues and problems with my gut. At first I had no clue what it was. At one point the cramps were so bad and wouldn't go away that I went to a doctor and did blood tests and a stool sample. I went on to suffer the symptoms and gut issues for perhaps two years. I'd heard of gluten intolerance, but I didn't know much about it–except that it was about people who had issues digesting wheat. Since I'd eaten wheat my whole life with no problem or issues at all, I never considered for a moment that I could have such a thing. So, I really had no interest in learning about the topic.

One day I stumbled upon an article about gluten intolerance and I think some symptoms listed in the catchy headline caught my attention. As I read through the article and they mentioned the symptoms and effects, I realized I was experiencing nearly all of them. I was pretty sure at that point that I indeed had gluten intolerance, but I of course wanted to be sure. So, I just informally took note of when I ate bread, pasta, etc. and how I felt afterwards. I compared it to days I didn't eat any gluten. I also intentionally stayed away from it for several days. Sure enough, the symptoms and issues were directly related to me eating gluten.

Now I'm a pretty intellectual guy and enjoy figuring things out. In the preceding years I had done a fair amount to educate myself about health, nutrition, and picked up some Biochemistry along the way. I've dealt with a number of health issues in the past by studying them and finding solutions to them, which usually entailed certain nutrients, herbs, or a combination of them. Oftentimes I discover causes or things to stay away from. In general, I usually arrive at a "stop doing this and start doing that" approach that worked. By the way, this general approach works in many areas of life as well.

I'm also a computer guy and good at internet research. So it was natural for me to decide that I needed to begin by fully understanding this gluten thing, and then find out what the solution to it was. I mean I certainly didn't want to live with the symptoms and discomfort, and I sure as heck didn't want to stop eating bread–not to mention all the other gluten containing foods like pasta or pizza.

However, as I first began researching I wasn't at all impressed with what I encountered. It seemed to me there wasn't too much understanding of the topic and there was something even worse: basically everyone just said the only thing to do was to stop eating gluten. I guess the logic is rather simple: don't eat it and you won't experience the effects or consequences. However, that was clearly insufficient and lame to me. I immediately realized that that advice is merely avoidance and eliminating symptoms; It is not actually fixing the problem or root cause. I basically thought to myself, "There is no way I'm going to stop eating gluten for the rest of my life; I'm going to dig into this and find out what the actual problem is and a way to actually fix it."

Well, I'm happy to report that I was apparently successful in doing just that. I'm convinced that I got to the root cause (and several contributing causes), and also found the solution(s). I then came up with a strategy to implement these and took the actions required. I fixed my gluten intolerance and can now eat it again without any issues. I think that you can achieve the same results by doing what worked for me: fully understand the problem and its causes, and then use my strategy to fix it. That is both why I wrote this book and also the main contents of it.

Chapter 3: What are Gluten Intolerance Symptoms?

If you are reading this book it is a fair bet that you are already aware of what "gluten intolerance" or "gluten sensitivity" does to you body and the side-affects or symptoms of it are. However, you may not be aware of the full list, or you may be using this book to get relief from some other health issue. It is also possible you are thinking, "maybe I have it, I think I do, but want to know more". Perhaps it is true that you believe suffer from it when you do not–that it is actually something else going on. Therefore, it is probably a good idea to discuss the symptoms and what it is typically like for a person that has "gluten intolerance".

But first, a bit more about the possibility that you (and others) believe they have it when actually they do not. Firstly, about 33% of Americans currently avoid or do not eat gluten. One would think they would do this only if they are gluten intolerant. However, some think it is just "bad for you", and there may be some truth to this we will discuss later. Others may be doing it because they think it will help them lose weight. Still others may have a few, or even many, of the symptoms and thus assume they have it when they actually do not.

Consider a study of 400 people that was referenced in Medical News Today. These people had self-diagnosed gluten intolerance: it turned out that 26 people had celiac disease, 2 had a wheat allergy, and only 27 of the remaining 364 people were diagnosed as gluten sensitive. That means that of the 400 who thought they were gluten intolerant, only 55 people (14.5%) actually had an issue with gluten. So it is highly likely they had the symptoms, but there was actually another cause for them. For example, irritable bowel syndrome has nearly identical symptoms–at least going gluten free actually helps a bit with this. Another example is FODMAP sensitivity, which are short-chain carbohydrates found in many foods, including wheat–people with this are better off to avoid FODMAPs and can actually eat gluten.

In summary of these points, having an accurate diagnosis of gluten intolerance/sensitivity isn't actually easy and straightforward. We will address what I think is a very good diagnosis approach later on.

Let's get back to the symptoms. Here is a laundry list: diarrhea, constipation, smelly feces, stomach cramps/pain, bloating, tiredness, headaches, skin problems, unexplained weight loss, joint/muscle pain, iron deficiency/anemia, arm/leg numbness, brain fog, anxiety, and depression. Probably the most common ones are this short list: diarrhea, stomach pains, tiredness, and depression.

There isn't a very good straight and simple answer in terms of how and when these symptoms manifest and what gluten intolerance is like for most people. Part of the reason for this is that each person's particular level of sensitivity is different, and so too is the absorption rate of their intestines and the time to impact–which can also be affected by the condition and/or root cause and culprit. What I mean by this last sentence is two-fold: the overall gut (lower intestine) health of each person varies as does the thickness of the lining–these impact the rate of absorption; the likely culprit we will discuss is degenerating gut health and so the more and longer someone has been a victim of it will determine response time and severity.

All of these variable aside, it can be pretty common to have the stomach go a bit haywire and get all grumpy 20-30 minutes after eating a gluten-rich meal. These can last a while, but typically fade as digestion is complete and perhaps after 2-6 hours. Diarrhea is typically experienced the next morning as this is a fairly regular time to eliminate and about on schedule for the previous days intake to work its way through. But, diarrhea may last for several days after just one gluten meal. On the other hand (likely for people with relatively healthier guts), it may take 2 to 5 days to even manifest side effects and have other symptoms. These factors combined can make it a bit tricky for people to initially realize symptoms are related to having eaten gluten. Note: we will later discover why it may take days for symptoms to manifest or to persist even though it would seem that all the gluten would be eliminated in a maximum of 24 hours.

Also, consider that many of the things on the list of symptoms are things that most people have from time to time. I mean, in today's world who the heck isn't frequently tired? Who among us doesn't get depressed occasionally? Everyone is going to have some stomach issues and diarrhea from time to time–perhaps eating something that just doesn't agree with you, too spicy, or eating too much fruit at a time. So it is having multiple symptoms and having them very regularly, near constantly, and in relation to having eaten gluten that is what is important to consider. It is also unfortunate that from the long laundry list of symptoms, most people don't have quite a number of the items listed.

Chapter 4: Why Fix your Gluten Sensitivity?

Why should you or anyone want to fix gluten sensitivity? There are the obvious reasons and ones already mentioned: the symptoms or side effects are uncomfortable, unpleasant, and annoying; if you don't want to suffer them then avoiding gluten means you can't eat breads, pastas, crackers, and tons of other great foods you likely enjoy and are a part of so many meals and types of cuisine.

Beyond this, avoiding gluten means having to do two other things that really stink: being a careful and informed shopper that has to have "gluten free", which can often cost a lot more; being careful or very restricted when eating out or at family/social gatherings, occasions, holidays, etc.

But there are actually more reasons beyond these perhaps obvious ones of which people suffering from gluten intolerance are already aware. Before I go into that specifically, let me approach it generally.

Symptoms of anything, but in particular health related symptoms, are occurring because there is some underlying problem, condition, or something messed up. Now if you treat a symptom you can make the symptom go away, but that doesn't fix the problem does it? Should you care if the problem is fixed as long as you don't have to deal with or feel the unpleasant symptom(s)?

Let's take a few examples to explore this a bit. Let's say you get a headache. So, you pop a pain reliever. The headache goes away. Problem solved, right? Wrong. Symptom alleviated is all. Sure the headache (symptom) went away, but what if it was caused from too much stress (actual problem)? Well, the issue with this approach is that you just pop those pain relievers every time you get a headache and never address the real problem of being over-stressed. It is a well-known fact that "stress is a killer" and is incredibly harmful to your health. In fact, "stress management" is included as one of the "four pillars of health". So, if you just pop that pill and treat the symptom of the headaches, something like heart disease, stroke, heart attack, and/or death may result years later due to the ongoing and cumulative effects of stress.

Now let's say you address the actual stress problem. Maybe you learn and practice some meditation, take some time for yourself and a hot bath in the evenings, take more time/days off work, reduce your workload and demands upon you by getting some help or simplifying, etc. Maybe you do a variety of things to reduce and manage stress–you end up living a long life and not having those horrible diseases or premature death. Seems like a good idea to deal with the actual problem instead of just getting rid of symptoms. So, as to that previous question: yes, you probably should care if the problem is fixed even if you don't have to deal with or feel the symptoms.

Here's another example. Let's say that when you drive your car that one day you discover that when you push down your gas pedal a bit fast and far that your engine sputters and the power is reduced. But, you figure out that if you push it down slowly and don't put on too much gas that it doesn't do this. Are you then going to just address this symptom using the gas pedal that way? Suppose it is happening because your fuel injectors are clogged up and so is your air filter. When months later you take a long trip you find your car finally breaks down and won't run at all–leaving you stranded on the side of the road. The mechanic in town says you need entirely new fuel injectors that cost one arm and three legs. As it turns out, you could have used injector cleaner and a new air filter for $40 when the symptoms first appeared. Avoidance of the problem and masking symptoms didn't help at all. In fact, avoiding problems by covering up or making symptoms go away can often lead to both the problems getting bigger as well as leading to other problems.

Perhaps another health example makes the point more clear. What if you are having hip pain and so you decide to take ibuprofen for it? Sure, that makes the pain go away and you are then treating only the symptom (pain and inflammation), but haven't addressed the real and underlying problem. You might keep doing this and have the hip get worse and worse. Since it hurts if you walk too much or run, then you avoid those activities. Let's suppose that eventually this leads to weight gain, high blood pressure, and then eventually to a hip replacement.

Now let's imagine that the problem was that the hip was simply out of place and/or some tight muscles were pulling it out of alignment. If instead of trying to treat/avoid the symptom you had investigated this and addressed it, then we could imagine a whole different outcome. Perhaps some physical therapy, deep tissue massage, chiropractic care, etc. would have put the hip back in place and stopped the tight muscles pulling it out. Since you fixed the problem, it then didn't go on over time to wear out the cartilage and end up grinding bone-on-bone. No hip replacement would have been needed. In this example we can also see how quality of life was decreased (not being able to walk much, run, enjoy being pain free) as well as it leading to other problems like the high blood pressure and weight gain.

So the points here are that treating/avoiding symptoms alone and not fixing the root problem is basically a flawed and unwise approach: it decreases the full range of experiences and can often lead to a problem getting worse. Important also is that problems in the body that are left untreated often create new and other problems because the body's system are so inter-connected and inter-dependant. The old saying of, "A stitch in time saves nine" applies here.

But there is still another point of why making symptoms go away is unwise. In terms of our bodies, symptoms are our body's way of trying to get our attention and tell us something is wrong. Symptoms such as pain, discomfort, inflammation, etc. are messages. The body might be saying, "Hey, I need to rest those muscles and recover", or "I need to be stretched", or "I'm allergic to or don't like that type of food", or "I have an injury here and you need to not use this for a while so I can heal." If we ignore the messages and make them go away, then we don't understand what the root problem to be fixed is.

Worse still, by eliminating the symptoms, we stop getting reminders/messages and so we don't pay attention or take actions. You may have heard the old expression, "The squeaky wheel gets the oil/grease", which usually means complaining and making a big fuss gets more attention and action than remaining quiet. Here I am meaning to suggest that symptoms are your body making a squeaky wheel to ensure you pay attention and do something about it. If you eliminate the squeaks then you do not have the continual reminder that serves to rather demand/scream that you need to take action and fix the problem.

Here's a quick example of how this works. I've had some back problems due to an injury. When it is hurting I know that doing stretches and physical therapy makes it better. So, I do those and sure enough it improves. Invariably then I stop doing the exercises because I'm not getting the reminder and I'm not being forced by the pain (message/symptom) to keep paying attention and keep taking action. After a while it starts hurting again and the cycle repeats. I used to think I'd learn my lesson and stay with it regularly, but alas we are forgetful beings and there are many demands for our time and attention as well as what seem higher priorities.

Now let's briefly mention how this unwise approach of eliminating symptoms specifically relates to gluten intolerance. In short, you have a problem in your gut! If you just avoid gluten to get rid of the symptoms, this gut problem is only going to get worse. It also can, and likely will, lead to multiple other health issues. These might include ones like irritable bowel syndrome, leaky gut syndrome, nutrient deficiencies, etc. These in turn can adversely affect other systems of the body and create other health issues. Again, you need to understand that the body is a highly complex and integrated system; It is rather like links in a chain; Each part of the system needs to do its job well in order to feed and support other systems. When one starts having problems and is breaking down, the next link in the chain suffers and then it eventually breaks down.

I said above "In short you have a problem with your gut." because we haven't covered the actual problem yet. After we have covered that, and in the end of Chapter 7, I will come back to remind you about the point of this short chapter: it is really important and there are good reasons to actually fix the problem and not just try to avoid gluten so you don't experience the symptoms. But I wanted to have this short chapter here to set the stage and give you some notion of how and why it is a good idea (wise) to actually fix your gluten intolerance that is beyond the obvious reasons already mentioned and that you already know.

I also want to tie back into what we discussed in the last chapter and that study of 400 self-diagnosed people. Recall that only 14.5% of them actually had gluten intolerance–at least according to the doctor's diagnosis. Now if we consider this in terms of the point of this chapter–fixing the problem–this means these people were likely making two errors: avoiding gluten to only prevent/avoid symptoms; not actually discovering what the problem really was.

Later on we will discuss our "likely culprit" and what creates the problem. Along the way we will also discover a few "contributing factors/culprits". With all of that information, and last chapter's laundry list of symptoms, I will explain a way to make a more accurate diagnosis. It is an approach that I think is better than the standard one.

Additionally, it is also the procedure to diagnose you will be doing to fix gluten intolerance, so it will be doing both of these in one fell swoop. Put another way, it will help you correctly diagnose and know if you have it, and if you do then you are well on your way to fixing it. If you don't then you will at least have found out and that might be really important so you can investigate other things and identify your actual problem.

Chapter 5: Understanding Gluten and Gliadin

So, what the heck is this "gluten" stuff anyway? Likely the general public, and even people with gluten sensitivity, don't actually know what gluten is. Some may have no idea at all, others may know just a little bit such as, "Well, it's some type of stuff in wheat." Perhaps some people have a bit more understanding such as "A type of protein in wheat and a few other grains." But as I said in the beginning, you need a fuller knowledge of it than that. This will be key to being able to understand what is going on in your body and also understanding both the real problem and the solution.

So let's get the "textbook" version and definition of what gluten is, which varies a bit depending upon the sources you research. Here is a short and simple definition:

Gluten is a general name for a group/family of proteins that are found in the endosperm of certain grains.

Now then, let's explain that a bit further and then delve into some details. That "endosperm" is a type of tissue produced in the plant seeds that helps their embryos when the plant germinates. It is like a big package of hundreds of proteins that gives the embryo everything they need to grow for a while. In a way, it is like the plant's version of an egg, which also has all the nutrients the embryo needs to grow into a chick–the reason eggs are so healthy for us to eat. So this pack of protein may have a lot of good stuff for us in it too–but perhaps not as we aren't wheat seeds. That it comes from this endosperm tissue is why gluten comes only from certain grains/seed plants.

Now that we know that much, a brief tangent fits here. Since it only comes from a number of grains, this is why tons of things in the supermarket are just marketing trying to get you to buy their brand. I mean I've actually seen "Gluten Free!" stickers on packages of bacon! Gluten doesn't come from and isn't in any type of meat, so these companies are preying upon a widespread ignorance of what gluten even is, and where it comes from. I've seen all sorts of "Gluten Free!" marketing on products that can't have gluten in the first place–it isn't like they are making some special version that is gluten free. What they are doing is to try to get ignorant consumers to buy their brand because it is "Gluten Free!" and imply that their competitor's products do have gluten in them.

Now there are lots of processed foods that have gluten in them and some companies that are making versions without it, so those labels make sense. There are also processing plants that make/refine multiple products in the same facility or even with the same machines. A prime example of this is oats. Oats don't have gluten in them. However, many brands are made in places where they process wheat or even barley. This can make something like gluten dust or residue that can end up in small amounts in the oats. Even for people with gluten sensitivity this is too little to be an issue. But for people with Celiacs disease this is a major problem because even trace amounts of gluten are big trouble for them. So, technically all oats are "Gluten Free!" until they get contaminated. If and when you aren't eating gluten, you don't need to concern yourself with oats or buy the special gluten free ones that are really for people with Celiacs. Note: some farmers do use glyphosate as a "desiccant" on oat crops–we will cover its use as a desiccant later, but there may be some residue on some oats due to this practice.

"Celiac's disease" will come up several more times in this book. Many people are unfamiliar with it, so a brief definition is in order. First of all, it is often written and referred to as simply "Celiacs" or "Celiac" as well. Here is the definition from the Celiac Disease Foundation: Celiac disease is a serious autoimmune disorder that can occur in genetically predisposed people where the ingestion of gluten leads to damage in the small intestine."

They go on to say, "It is estimated to affect 1 in 100 people worldwide. Two and one-half million Americans are undiagnosed and are at risk for long-term health complications. When people with celiac disease eat gluten (a protein found in wheat, rye and barley), their body mounts an immune response that attacks the small intestine. These attacks lead to damage on the villi, small fingerlike projections that line the small intestine, that promote nutrient absorption. When the villi get damaged, nutrients cannot be absorbed properly into the body. Celiac disease is hereditary, meaning that it runs in families."

So, you can think of Celiac as gluten sensitivity on steroids, or a really severe, genetically based version of it. The notable differences are that for people with Celiac, even tiny amounts of gluten cause major reactions and the primary issue is that their autoimmune system attacks their small intestine. For people that just have gluten intolerance/sensitivity, that immune response and attack on the intestine does not occur. Note: later we will discover data that shows that Celiac disease was quite rare 20 years ago, but has been skyrocketing ever since. So, that estimate mentioned of 1 in 100 people is a current one and shouldn't be taken to mean this has always been a rather common or prevalent disease.

Where were we before that tangent? Oh yeah, delving into the definition of gluten. Okay, so it is a bunch of proteins in grains. Now we are all familiar with the word "protein", but do we really know what it is and means? You might know just a little such as, "Well, it's the stuff in meat, fish, dairy, nuts, and beans that is good for building muscles."

Well, they said gluten is a general name for proteins, but it turns out "proteins" is actually a general name too–it is like saying "meat" without specifying if it is chicken, beef, deer, fish, etc. "Protein" is a general name referring to various amounts and arrangements of what are called amino acids. It mainly refers to many of these amino acids basically stuck or strung together into long chains in a variety of forms or configurations at the molecular level.

For example, certain amino acids link together in short chains, some medium, some will branch off, some get very long, and they also mix and match different ones. In atypical scientific fashion they actually named these in a sensible way where the meaning is clear: short-chain, medium-chain, branched-chain, and long-chain amino acids. It is rather like having a LEGO set where you have a fixed number of different shaped pieces, but you can link and connect them together and use various ones to make a huge variety of constructions. The pieces are amino acids and the final large constructions are proteins.

So, you can have several amino acids bound together into a cluster or chain with a covalent bond, which they call a peptide. When the chains get really long they stop calling them peptides and call them proteins. This is likely for convenience sake and to avoid the complexity of having to identify and name all of the possible peptides. It is an arbitrary length, but it seems that over 50 links in the chain is when they start calling it a protein. In terms of the human body, when we eat these they get broken back apart–eventually down to just peptides and amino acids. We will go further into the details of this later.

For now just understand that nature does this construction of amino acid LEGO pieces and we get proteins as input to our bodies. Just as importantly, our body breaks them back apart into the base amino acid pieces and then is able to use them as the building blocks of many things and even to manufacture its own big proteins based upon its needs. This is why there are some "nonessential amino acids" because our body can use the other amino acids to construct them when it needs them. Technically there can be a limit to how many of some of these it can make at a time. When the body is very stressed or ill it may need you to eat these nonessential ones to make up the shortfall–these are called "conditional amino acids."

So, at the root level it all boils down to amino acids. Amino acids are technically organic compounds that have at least one amino group and one carboxy group–never mind that jargon. A simple understanding is that the amino group has Nitrogen and Hydrogen in it and the carboxy group has Carbon, Oxygen, and Hydrogen; These very basic and important elements are key ones composing many molecules based upon numbers and arrangements–for example you have what you need there to make water or carbon dioxide, etc.

What is important generally are a few things about amino acids: we know of 22 different kinds of amino acids relevant to humans; adult humans can only produce or build 13 of them within the body, so the other nine must be eaten. The amino acids that humans cannot produce internally are called "essential amino acids" because they are required for us to live and for the body to function. So they are "essential" to eat because you can't make them, and "essential" to have because without them you die.

Plants can make all of the amino acids and of course we can get them by eating plants. Though this doesn't mean that eating some plant will give you all of them, or in equal or healthy ratios. Animals, like us, also have them, and they are the main part of what makes up their muscles–so that is why eating meat gives us lots of protein (a variety of amino acids strung together into long chains).

Our bodies use amino acids to do more things than could be explained in an entire book–and likely many more things we don't even know about yet. But, they are so versatile and critically important that it is worth mentioning some. They are of course used to build muscles. But beyond that they are used for a lot of chemical signaling in the body, as an energy source after conversion to glucose, as building blocks for every cell membrane, to make energy in the mitochondria, making DNA/RNA, and to make very important things like hormones, insulin, enzymes, and neurotransmitters.

Basically most all of your body is made of these amazing chemical compounds or dependant upon them. Nearly every system of the body utilizes them in some form–think about the fact that you cannot even think without them. Add this bit of knowledge about amino acids to your repository so you know just how important protein is to your body and health. Also add in this tidbit: you cannot store up and save amino acids for later use like you can do with carbohydrates, fats, and many vitamins and minerals–you need to consume your amino acids (protein) each and every day–you don't have to eat them at each meal, but at some point cumulatively in a day.

Back to gluten then being a general name. Gluten is a whole family of proteins–perhaps more than 100. Since there are only 22 amino acids, we can deduce that most of these are then groups of amino acids chemically joined together into really long chains or into the shorter ones called peptides. But to simplify things for our needs, there really are two main categories, and also main amounts, of these proteins: glutenin (47%) and gliadin. It also contains 25% glutamic acid.

Now that we have drilled down a bit deeper, we need to find out what glutenin, gliadin, and glutamic acid are. We can simply consult the list of the 22 amino acids and apply some logic. Doing so we find out that gliadin is not listed and neither is glutenin. We do find glutamic acid listed as a non-essential. So, we can quickly realize that glutenin and gliadin must be peptides.

It turns out that what causes problems for many people is the gliadin. It also turns out there are three forms of this gliadin peptide and mainly one (and perhaps two) are the troublemakers. The troublemaker appears to be this alpha-gliadin peptide with a specific 33 amino acid sequence. So, we now know a bit more in detail what the problem area is related to: a 33 link chain of amino acids that is the alpha-gliadin peptide coming from the endosperm of certain grains.

Since we know that after we eat gliadin peptides our gut raises some ruckus and gets upset, it is rather obvious that something is going on with the digestive process of it. Therefore, we need to now shift over to digestion in order to continue delving into understanding what is going on here. After we understand digestion better and see the Chemistry of what is going on, we will bring back and briefly discuss gliadin peptides in particular.

The problem or issue isn't with "gluten" exactly. The issue is with one particular peptide in the gluten that is "alpha-gliadin-33" and something about how our digestive system handles and responds to it.

Chapter 6: Gliadin Digestion and Enzymes

In this chapter we are going to cover quite a lot of ground. We are going to delve into the digestion of the trouble-making alpha-gliadin-33. In order to do that, we are going to have to cover protein digestion generally. We will also explore a couple of other topics related to digestion and the small intestine as well. Some of this is going to get a bit technical, but I will do my best to keep it somewhat simple by using some metaphors and layman's terminology.

Additionally, I'll provide some summaries and simple language to ensure it is clear and understandable. Hopefully all of this combined will provide you with a sufficient level of understanding. But, I'm giving you a "heads-up" and just do your best to plough through this stuff because I do feel it is important. It may also help to re-read this chapter; Doing so will lead to it making more sense and getting a fuller understanding.

Likely and hopefully somewhere in your schooling you were taught the basics of human digestion. But, if you are anything like I am, that was a while ago and you forgot a lot. I don't want to go into a long and irrelevant review of it, but perhaps a very simple refresher particularly related to digesting protein will be helpful and appropriate. I will also include some tidbits that have a bearing and impact on protein and gliadin peptides.

So we get some protein and shove it in our mouths. We then chew it up. You may have done this little experiment in science class in about 7th grade where you used PH strips and chewed up a saltine cracker. You would chew it up just a little and test it, then chew it for like a minute and test it again. The PH strip showed you its acid/base level was changing, and this was meant to teach you about the acid/base science as well as the fact that you had digestive enzymes in your saliva that started the digestion process very early on in the your overall digestive system and tract.

This is all fine and well, but a cracker is a carbohydrate and not a protein or big chunk of amino acids. So there aren't actually any enzymes in your saliva that go to work breaking down protein. In terms of meat however, at least you have made the big hunk/bite a lot smaller by chewing it, and that certainly is a start. But keep in mind that those amino acids are microscopic and very tiny molecules–and that is what you eventually need to break the protein apart into in order to make use of it. Point being this chewed up stuff is still "huge" in digestive terms.

Next we swallow the protein and it hits the stomach. Since you likely haven't eaten in a while, your stomach has brewed up a nice batch of stomach acid (hydrochloric acid) that the swallowed blob of protein (called a bolus) is plunged into. Also, when food starts hitting the stomach it releases a bunch more acid it has made just for the occasion. Now this hydrochloric acid is powerful stuff. So, it can take these still relatively big chunks and dissolve them down quite a bit. It does what Chemists often do with alcohol or acids: denaturation. The stomach also contracts and massages the contents around like a washing machine on steroids.

Let's skip ahead a bit and then we will back up again–this will hopefully make more sense this way. Eventually this food is going to end up in your small intestine where it can get absorbed into the blood. The lining of the walls of the intestine is tissue called the epithelium, and the membrane is called the mucosa. Within this "lining" or "wall" of the small intestine are these little hair-like things on the folds called villi. These guys and the mucosa absorb all the nutrients and pass it into the blood.

Now the mucosa and villi only let very small things through; They are basically filtering out what has been digested and is usable (food) and what isn't digestible or usable (garbage/waste). So, only the single amino acids or short peptides that have only two or three amino acids (dipeptides and tripeptide) are transported in. Therefore, in order to absorb protein it must be completely digested and broken down into these incredibly small molecules. Just the stomach acid and churning can't do that, so we need something to help out.

Now then, we already know these proteins arrived in much longer chains where they had these chemical bonds holding them together. So, what we need to make them small enough to absorb is something that fits in there like a key and opens the locks of these chemical bonds to break apart the chains. Well, it just so happens that we have just such a key, and this key is actually made of amino acids! This makes perfect sense since it is the same sort of molecule that can get in there and sort of mate with amino acids in the chain or dislodge them from the chain by a variety of techniques including forcing some water in there to break up the glue/bond at the linking points (hydrolysis). These vital little "keys" are called digestive enzymes.

Okay, let's jump back again. In the stomach then, the stomach acid triggers and activates multiple digestive enzymes generally. Since most of the proteins are peptides, they named the stomach's main protein-digesting enzyme pepsin. It goes to work by breaking the peptide bonds that hold the molecules together–sort of like dissolving their glue or prying apart the LEGO pieces. Well it does the work it can in the time it has allowed, but things keep moving down and it can only break up so many types of bonds. It is a great worker that can withstand the very acidic stomach environment and is very generalized in terms of being able to work on a variety of peptides.

The food/protein then moves down the system. There are some details of bile being released and the acidic mixture being changed back to alkaline so it won't dissolve your intestines, but we can skip that stuff. Eventually then a sludge enters the first part of the small intestine and the pancreas gets signaled it needs to get involved and do its job. So the pancreas is going to help finish the job by excreting/dumping more enzymes in, which it made and stored in an inactive form. Those enzymes include these among others: trypsin, chymotrypsin, elastase, and carboxypeptidase.

The last one carboxypeptidase is one we can already mostly understand from the parts of the word we recognize. I'm sure you recalled amino acids have a "carboxy" group, right? Oh no wait, I think I said you could "never mind that jargon". The "pep" is again like "pepsin" and "peptide". So, we know that basically this enzyme is going to go target the carboxy group bonding points to break apart peptides. The very last part is "ase", and this is a very common and standard suffix that is added onto the names of enzymes (including also the enzymes we use to build proteins from amino acids). For example, the sugar lactose in milk is digested by the enzyme lactase, and sucrose by sucrase, etc.

In the blood of the cell walls of the intestine is another worker, aminopeptidase N, who also does some good finish work attacking the amino-terminal end of the peptides. There are also several types of aminopeptidase inside the cells that are inside the walls of the intestine, which have various specialties at breaking up different types of peptides and their bonds.

I've only mentioned the protein-digesting enzymes that are commonly discussed, but it should be noted that there are actually many more than these. Most of these many enzymes are doing very specialized work–certain ones break apart certain chain types that others cannot. Some use different attack strategies, attack points, and tools/weapons. So this whole host of enzymes working as a team finishes up the job started by pepsin and the stomach acid in the stomach.

Let's backup up just a bit, the aminopeptidases are rather unique because they aren't being excreted by the pancreas, but instead are actually residing inside the cells located within the wall/lining of the intestine itself. What if the intestine's epithelium, mucosa, and villi are somehow compromised or damaged? Perhaps the aminopeptidases would then not be present to do their important job, or maybe their numbers have been radically reduced.

Maybe the gliadin peptide is a tricky one to break apart generally. Maybe the gliadin peptides need to have their amino-terminal ends broken apart in order to be reduced to a single amino acid or a dipeptide or tripeptide. If that doesn't happen, they certainly can't be absorbed because they are too big. What does the body do when it has something it can't digest, absorb, and make use of? How does it respond? We will revisit these questions in a little while. For now, let's continue to the end of the digestion process.

Now that the protein has been broken down into small enough sizes, we go back to it being absorbed via the walls of the intestine and those villi guys. At that point the single amino acids and di/tri peptides go into the blood. From there all sorts of things happen to them including processing and changes being done to them by the liver, kidney, and elsewhere.

For example, the liver might take that glutamic acid and strip off just a single proton and turn it into glutamate, which the brain and nervous system use as the glutamate neurotransmitter as well as using it to make proteins it needs. I said, "might" because I don't know if that conversion is done by the liver, but it makes sense as the liver does many of these Chemistry conversions and also is signaled by the brain with something like "supply orders" to fulfill its needs. We do know the liver will convert glutamic acid into glutamine. At times, some amount of amino acids may need to be converted to glucose for energy, and certainly the liver does that. But, as we discussed earlier, these amino acids get used to do many things and in multiple areas of the body. So the point is we get them into the blood and they get circulated and used where and as needed.

I've tried to keep our review and summary of digestion simple, but there is a very important aspect of it I need to mention. Our endocrine system is involving and using hormones at each step in the digestive process; All the systems and parts of the process require these hormones. These hormones are the "messengers" that start things happening, stop them, and control/regulate them. Hormones trigger the release of the stomach acid, cause the dumping of bile, inform the pancreas to dump in the enzymes, and hormones are present and actively participate in the chemical reactions in the small intestine. We will discuss hormones more in the next chapter.

Let's again back up a bit and return to these villi guys. If you imaging your small intestine as just a hose or tube (technically the lumen is the open/inside part), you can realize it has a certain amount of surface area: the inner circumference multiplied by the length. So any foodstuffs going thru it can and must only be absorbed by it across this surface area. Now if the foodstuff slurry is moving through at a fairly constant rate, your body wants and needs to absorb as many nutrients as possible before it passes all the way out. More surface area for absorption would really help out here.

One thing done to increase surface area was to make folds in and out–instead of the inside being just a flat tube. But it turns out that even more area is required. That is precisely what the villi are for and do. You could imagine them as hairs sticking up all over the inner part of the tube (and the folds of it). Or you could picture them as straws sticking out at all sorts of angles on the inside of a pipe/tube. Since they are doing absorbing too, and actually the majority of it, this radically increases the overall surface area for absorption of nutrients.

Again this raises some questions and possible concerns. Are these villi guys invulnerable? Can they be compromised, destroyed, or just die of old age? Obviously if they get trashed, killed off, or messed up then we can't absorb our nutrients, which is going to cause all sorts of havoc and issues. Since their health is so important, what harms them and what do they require to be healthy?

Well, it turns out they are quite fond of a peptide called glutamine. No, that is not the same as glutanin that comes with our gluten (I knew that you caught that and were paying attention). Glutamine is used by the villi to maintain their health and structural integrity–if they are Popeye, then it is their spinach. So it sounds like good and important stuff. Where and how do we get it?

Glutamine is made by doing a small conversion on glutamate, which again is basically glutamic acid except minus one proton. This conversion is done by cells lining the intestinal tract. Well now isn't that handy? This means it can basically be made "on site" and supplied right to the villi. It can also be made by the liver and the kidneys. But, there are some potential issues here. Again, what if the lining of the intestine is damaged? That would mean those cells couldn't make and supply the glutamine/spinach to the villi–and we know that spells big trouble if they are compromised since we need them to absorb our nutrients.

Another issue is that unfortunately a few of the foods highest in the glutamic acid/glutamate have something about them that actually damages the villi as well. I'm sure you recall that gluten has lots of glutamic acid in it–25%. It seems wheat is particularly hard on our villi, and that is a bummer, but it also turns out it is supplying the perfect thing to repair the damage it does. One can wonder if it helps as much as it hurts, or hurts more than it helps. Other foods that apparently do a number on and trash our villi include corn, soy, and casein (a protein in dairy). However, these are all high in glutamic acid as well.

I'm not sure why these particular 4 hurt our villi. I wonder about the high fiber content of the wheat, soy, and corn: normally we like fiber because it basically scrapes and cleans the walls of our colon (large intestine); but before it can do this it is passing through our small intestine. As it does this, does it also scrape or nearly shave off the villi? We will revisit this later on when we discuss giving your small intestine a "time out to heal" via brief fasting.

Now one can start to wonder if a persons overall diet can be doing things that have compromised the small intestine and thus impaired several important processes of digesting proteins. So far we see a potential for damage to compromise one of our protein-digesting enzyme groups, aminopeptidases that live in the plasma inside the cells inside the intestine walls. We also are making glutamine in the very same place, which our villi need. Additionally, we might be eating too much of some foods that trash our villi: wheat, corn, soy, and dairy.

It isn't hard to imagine that perhaps wheat gives enough help/healing to the villi via the high amount of glutamic acid it contains. But maybe our intestine walls, mucosa, and the villi aren't fairing so well due to other things we are consuming. It seems illogical that just the wheat is doing the harm/damage. Recall my personal story of all that bread I ate growing up–and this story is common for many people. I also ate lots of cheese, and I drank milk with nearly every meal–as was common and recommended back then. Again this begs the question, "How could I eat like that for decades and never have any problem?" It seems rather obvious there must be more to the story and something else going on. If our gut is somehow broken or damaged, then it seems there is some other thing(s) that are harming and degrading its functioning.

Since we now have covered the entire digestion and absorption process of protein, let's first summarize in layman's terms and then look at "after absorption". Then we will move on to some related topics.

Digestion of protein simplified is this: chewing it up; dissolving it with stomach acid and one enzyme in the stomach; then finishing the job of breaking up the very long chains into single or tiny molecules called amino acids in the small intestine using a whole team/group of enzymes; most of these are thrown into the mix by the pancreas, but a few are doing their work in the wall of the intestine itself; once fully digested they are absorbed through the intestine wall and enter the blood stream. The endocrine system (hormones) is a key part of controlling nearly every part of the digestive process.

Now let's move on to after absorption. We can generalize our review of digestion and realize that in similar ways every type of food, vitamin, and other nutrient get into our bodies at the very end of the process/cycle by the gut (small intestine). If there is some problem going on with the small intestine or digestion being accomplished there, then we can't get our nutrients–amino acids, carbohydrates, fats/lipids, vitamins, and minerals. If we imagine not getting these even when we are eating enough, or getting very little absorption of them, then some consequences should be rather obvious.

Since we can use protein, fats, and/or carbs for energy, then we would have a very low energy supply. Also, the B vitamins are essential for energy conversions. Both of these would mean that we would be tired a lot. Since we would basically be eating but not getting the value and absorption of the food, it would really be like not eating at all. What happens when you don't eat at all? Right, weight loss. Since we need amino acids to make our neurotransmitters and hormones, we might suspect our brain would be affected and have imbalances that might give it a headache and our hormones going out of whack may affect our moods and make us have trouble sleeping, irritability, or even depression.

Hmm, is this list of consequences at all familiar? It should be, it is the main list of symptoms of gluten intolerance/sensitivity. A potential point here is that really these symptoms may actually all be the result of non-absorption of nutrients, deficiencies, and basically malnutrition. As further supportive evidence, the list of symptoms of amino acid deficiency is also nearly identical. This suggests that what is really going on is a fundamental problem in the small intestine and non-absorption of proteins/amino acids generally–and potentially other nutrients as well. We will just consider this as a possible theory.

Again I remind you that the human body is a complex system composed of inter-connected and inter-dependant sub-systems. When one of these goes haywire, there is a trickle-down or cascading affect on the rest. In terms of the body, the very first thing in the system is the digestive system and absorption process because this is the input and supplies what every part and other system of the body relies upon. The only thing that is prior to this is either outside the body or at the very beginning of it: what we choose to stuff into the mouth, which is the first input point, but that is not really a system of the body. I found this Ayurvedic proverb that fits here and the previous point made about our food choices may be impacting our villi and gut health generally:

Last chapter we delved into gluten and got down into the alpha-gliadin-33 bugger. Now that we have covered protein digestion, absorption and after absorption, let's see what in particular goes on with gliadin that is making such a ruckus in our guts. I will spare you the rather complex Biochemistry of digesting gluten peptides and gliadin for two reasons: the complexity won't help you, and I'm no expert. I'm not sure I understand it fully myself, nor confident I would explain it correctly.

They key thing to understand as simplistically summarized is this: It turns out that the gluten proteins are in the same family/type as proline (an amino acid). This family is called prolamins. Also there is lots of proline in the gluten proteins. This proline stuff has a side chain sticking off it that makes it very rigid and strong–it is a tough guy. There is also something about how it doesn't want to play nice and do hydrogen bonding with others–this may lead to it being tough to hydrolyze or be broken up by other tactics.

Now here is where the real rub comes in. As the family of gluten proteins (prolamins) are being digested, we sort of end up with this leftover proline residue soup. This residue and the proline turn out to actually affect gliadin's structure that is next to and around it. Basically they make the gliadin really strong and rigid. Imagine a loose pile of iron filings that you can easily move around or blow away (weak). Now imagine putting a magnet under them so they form the structure of the magnetic flux lines and become fixed, structured, and rigid (strong and you can no longer blow them away/apart). This is what the proline and its residue do to the gliadin peptide; It makes them stronger and tough/impossible for the enzymes to break apart; the proline soup therefore makes gliadin peptides resistant to the enzymes doing their job. It should be noted that it is known that the enzymes do partially break down the alpha-gliadin.

The bottom line is that most of the protein in gluten is broken down sufficiently small (digested) and is absorbed. However, this tough bugger alpha-gliadin-33-mer peptide doesn't get broken down all the way and/or not all of it gets broken down because it gets beefed up by the proline stuff that thwarts the work of the enzymes. Metaphorically, the proline stuff turns the gliadin into Superman and our enzyme bullets just bounce off its chest. The result is that the partially digested alpha-gliadin peptides end up floating around in the small intestine. Since they are made of over 10 amino acids joined together in length, these are what are generally known as oligopeptides.

While I said they end up floating around, and that is likely true, very technical papers I have read also indicate they will enter into cells in the intestine's wall, but maybe they don't get absorbed and make it into the blood because they are too big. Remember that there are those enzymes (aminopeptidases) inside the cell's plasma that put on some final touches of breaking down the peptides. What may be happening is the gliadin oligopeptides basically get stuck in the cells or lining of the intestine, and this may be exactly what is causing the pain, cramps, etc.

By analogy, it is like cutting up a big piece of steak on your plate into bite-sized pieces. The knife represents your digestive enzymes. While the gliadin does get cut up into a smaller chunk, that chunk is still too big to fit in your mouth or swallow–so it is too big to get absorbed by the villi and wall of the small intestine. It sort of sits on the plate and rots or if you try to swallow it you gag and spit it out– treated as a toxin and an inflammatory response occurs. Some of it you try to swallow and it gets stuck in your throat and you choke–stuck inside the cells of the intestine's wall.

You may recall from our discussion of symptoms that they can manifest or last even 2-4 days after eating gluten and I said we would later discover why this is–despite that it should have been pooped out long before then. So, this then is the answer–they get embedded inside the intestine itself. Also, I think the pain wouldn't occur if the oligopeptides were just floating through the soup in the intestine tube (lumen) because it wouldn't be in contact enough with the nerves to do that. We might imagine the cramps and pain is due to the large alpha-gliadin oligiopeptides wedging themselves in-between epithelial cells and the walls to stretch it like a balloon.

Sources about Celiac disease claim these gliadin oligopeptides are actually toxic. For a person with Celiac disease, they trigger an immune response, which in turn attacks the gut itself as a basically misidentified invasion. Obviously they are "toxic" to those with Celiacs. Their immune system may be attacking the intestine itself due to the alpha-gliadin stuck inside the cells in the intestine walls–they see the entire intestine as something like a toxin, virus, bacteria, or foreign body/invader.

For people without Celiac disease, this autoimmune response doesn't occur, but certainly an inflammatory response occurs which is why the symptoms of bloating, cramps, stomach pain, etc. happen. Basically the stomach is saying, "Since I can't digest this stuff fully it must not be food and good for me; Therefore it is a toxin. What the heck is this crap you put in me? I don't want it. Get it out. I can't seem to get most of it out, so I better call for inflammation to get some white blood cells and circulation in here; I should also send a pain signal so my owner knows something is wrong down here with my intestinal lining."

Generally speaking this is what your body always says and does when you put stuff in it that isn't something it can digest and use. If for example you swallowed some lighter fluid then it would identify it as "non-usable food" and stimulate a response to make you vomit. It of course does the same thing if you drink too much alcohol, which of course is technically a poison. If you eat contaminated food, you get food poisoning and your body will first try to make you vomit, and the next morning you will likely have diarrhea, as it wants to flush out any leftovers as fast as possible. If you sprain you ankle it swells up (inflammation). Inflammation is a double-edged sword. It can at first bring in blood flow and white blood cells to combat infection. However, it can also then restrict blood flow at the site and to other areas; It can also restrict mobility in a way that healing is slower and not done properly. Due to the inter-connected nature of the body, inflammation that may help one area/system may adversely impact another. Previously I had asked what happens if the body can't digest something or has a problem and said we would discuss it later; This is that "later". In short, it nearly always has an inflammatory response— most gluten intolerance/sensitivity symptoms are the results of inflammation. While a little bit of inflammation for a brief time isn't a bad thing, it is well known that chronic inflammation is a serious health issue with many negative impacts.

We have just covered a big chunk of information. So, let's pause here to summarize. If you want to impress your friends and co-workers with your newfound knowledge and appear very intelligent, you could say something like this, which is a technical summary of what we have covered thus far:

There really isn't such a thing as "gluten sensitivity". Gluten contains hundreds of proteins and peptides that are no problem at all. What people really have is a problem fully digesting the alpha-gliadin-33-mer peptide due to how proline residue makes it resistant to the proteolytic enzymes secreted by the pancreas in the small intestine as well as the aminopeptidases inside the epithelium cell's blood serum. This lack of complete digestion leads the body to identify the undigested alpha-gliadin oligopeptides as toxins, which then stimulates an inflammatory response and other responses to rid its self of them and bring help to bear on the situation.

There is some chance that by now you actually understand to some degree just what all that jargon means. I would venture to say that you also now understand gluten intolerance better than 99% of people, and we haven't even delved into the rest of the story!

Let's discuss digesting gluten generally some more. Gluten is known to be a very strong group of proteins generally. It is sort of like a bunch of rubber bands stuck together with thick flexible glue. It is for this reason that the gluten in bread is so great for making bread. The gluten in the wheat flour makes the dough strong, yet flexible. When yeast is added and the bread rises, air pockets and bubbles form. The gluten keeps these bubbles from bursting and the dough from collapsing. Put another way, without the gluten the air bubbles would form, grow, and then pop; You would be left with something like a flat bread that is hard, tough and more like trying to eat a piece of cardboard. Indeed, many types of bread made from non-gluten grains turn out just like this–and have been made and eaten for thousands of years. So a piece of bread that has gluten in it turns into a final product that is light, soft, and chewy. Basically modern man ate it and said, "Now this is some darn good bread!"

The importance here is that gluten is fundamentally a tough and strong protein tangle, and that structure and strength makes it harder to digest compared to other proteins that, relatively speaking, are soft and not very strong.

My research also dug up what may be another important nugget of information. Apparently and supposedly, the proteins in gluten also stimulate the release of a chemical called zonulin. This chemical controls the bond between cells and regulates intestinal permeability (how thick/thin it is and how much gets through it), or its relative "leakiness". So, the more gluten proteins we eat, the more zonulin is released, and the intestinal wall gets more leaky. This would then be true for everyone regardless of having Celiac disease or gluten sensitivity. I do not know why this happens, but it may be that the zonulin is trying to open the cells up to receive the glucemic acid so that they can make the glutamine that the villi need for their health. Unfortunately this is happening at the same time the big alpha-gliadin oligopeptides are present and allows them to get taken/wedge in as well. This would seem to make sense.

If the gluten then triggers the zonulin release, this would mean that in general eating gluten, or at least too much of it, may actually be compromising our intestines. However, it should be understood that "leaky gut" isn't the same as getting things absorbed into the blood, but rather that it basically leaks outside into the entire cavity surrounding the gut. This means that "yucky" stuff that we would normally eliminate in our feces gets inside our body as occurs in leaky gut syndrome–not a good thing. It would also mean that good nutrients are leaking and are therefore not being absorbed–instead of the walls and villi absorbing them, they pass between the cells and leak out. This supports the previously mentioned general approach of not eating too much gluten regardless, and that moderation is the key.

Summarizing what we have learned, we now know that it actually may be impossible for our digestive enzymes to fully digest alpha-gliadin peptides. They are really strong/tough peptides to begin with, and also get resistant to our enzymes due to the proline and its residue. That incomplete digestion causes our body to identify them as toxic (and some claim they actually are toxins in that form). This in turn causes our body to have an inflammatory response, which generates many of the symptoms of "gluten sensitivity". Some of these undigested peptides may actually become embedded/stuck in the wall of our intestine. Additionally, there may be other things compromising the general health and absorption capabilities of our small intestines such that many symptoms are actually occurring due to nutrient deficiencies. One of these other things could be that eating gluten releases zonulin and makes our intestinal walls thin and leaky. To minimize and mitigate all of these things, a general approach of eating gluten in moderation seems wise.

But, if our protein-digesting enzymes fundamentally can't digest alpha-gliadin, then how were so many of us able to eat wheat for so many years without having any problem? You are probably asking, "Is there perhaps some other way to digest it other than by using enzymes?" Or more generally, "Is there another way we digest besides stomach acid and enzymes?"

What a great question! I'm so glad you asked. Most people aren't aware of this interesting fact: the human body in and of itself is also incapable of digesting most all vegetables! Did you know that? Certainly they get digested, but it turns out it isn't our body doing it. So, what is digesting our vegetables? It turns out we have these wonderful little helpers that are actually foreign life forms that do it for us. They are something between a parasite and a friend. They do feed off us, but we also get many benefits as well (this is called parasitic symbiosis).

They are often called your "gut flora". They are a complex community of microorganisms that live in your digestive tract. Basically they are helpful bacteria. At about 1 to 2 years of age, this huge colony of them basically gets imbedded in the intestinal epithelium and the intestinal mucosa barrier. The colony and your small intestine actually then develop together and create a unified system. Your intestine sees them as friends or even part of itself, and the bacteria do the same and consider your gut their home or maybe even view you as their mother. I say mother because they end up getting fed, housed, and given a nurturing environment. In exchange, they actually do many very beneficial functions for us–including breaking down the tough cellulose of vegetables so we can get at the nutrients stored inside.

You have likely heard of probiotics. It is both another term for these helpful strains of bacteria also usually means that someone is taking them–like taking antibiotics. Taking probiotics is consuming billions of these helpful bacteria. Various strains of the bacteria are available and commonly used. In general, people taking probiotics are trying to increase the size of their colony, restore it, and ensure it is healthy because of all the good work they do. Since they are living bacteria, once the colony is populated and healthy, they will replicate and reproduce–unless we do something that kills them or starves them.

It is well known that antibiotics wipe a lot of them out. We take antibiotics to kill "bad bacteria", but they work indiscriminately and so they also kill our "good bacteria"–probiotics/gut flora. So, after taking antibiotics it is a very good idea to take a bunch of probiotics to restore your colony. Have you ever taken antibiotics? If so, did you then take probiotics and restore your colony? If you did not, then wouldn't you have a pretty lame and mostly dead gut flora system? If so, you might have trouble digesting and getting nutrients from vegetables. Also, you might have trouble digestion other things, as we will soon discuss.

Other things can compromise your colony as well. It is widely believed that the unbeneficial fungus/yeast candida can grow out of control and basically take over all the space, incoming food, and other resources–usually this is attributed to eating too many carbohydrates (which break down into sugar), sugar, and also alcohol consumption (which is very similar to sugar) because the candida thrive on sugar. When this happens, the variety of other helpful gut flora basically get starved to death and crowded out by the candida overgrowth.

The point here is that our gut flora actually do quite a bit of digestion for us. A University of León study found that gut bacteria of healthy volunteers were able to break down gluten proteins. So the answer to the question about another way to digest gluten and the solution to the riddle of "why all of the sudden now is gluten a problem" may be partially revealed:

Even though your own enzymes probably can't fully digest gluten (alpha-gliadin-33), your gut flora can–as long as you have a good healthy colony of them. It may be that your enzymes along with the gut flora can get the full job done. But if you lack a healthy colony of gut flora, then you may no longer be able to fully digest the alpha-gliadin peptides that cause so much trouble.

Now we are getting somewhere! Certainly a strategy to "Fix Gluten Sensitivity and Heal Your Gut" is going to involve boosting up our gut flora via lots of probiotics. Taking them in pill form (or even liquids) isn't the only alternative, but it is a good, effective and simple one. Many of these bacteria can be cultivated by fermentation. Whether you are aware of it or not, making and eating fermented foods is quite popular now for just this reason–ensuring the gut has a big, healthy colony of flora/helpful bacteria. Things like yogurt have them, so does sauerkraut, kambucha, and there are also grain kefirs and other ways to make kefirs (self-replicating colonies of good bacteria).

You can use kefirs as "starters" and make many types of fermented vegetables, yogurt, fermented coconut milk, etc. All of these homemade probiotics take some knowledge, time, and maintenance; The benefit is they are typically way cheaper than purchasing probiotics as supplements. That said, the supplements really aren't that expensive; They also may have more choice and options on a diversity of strains/types, which most everyone agrees is a good thing. They are likely similar to enzymes in that some are better at digesting certain things than others. Additionally, they do many other helpful functions and there can be specialties each strain has for these as well.

I also want to throw this tidbit in here because it may be very important. We've talked a lot about our protein-digesting enzymes. I mentioned these are made of amino acids. But I hadn't yet mentioned that in order for our enzymes to function we need a particular mineral: magnesium. In fact, magnesium is critically important and plays role in over 300 enzyme functions!

Magnesium has gotten a lot of attention in recent years because it is critically important to a wide variety of functions the body performs. Pretty much every source quotes the same statistic that at least 50% of Americans are magnesium deficient–some sources say this is as high as 80%. Now put the pieces together: magnesium deficiency means your digestive enzymes are not going to be working.

Therefore, it is quite logical that a component of gluten intolerance is actually at least partially caused by, or made worse by, magnesium deficiency–lacking enough magnesium, your protein-digesting enzymes can't do their job very well, and in terms of gliadin it is already a very tough job!

In terms of gluten sensitivity, the standard advice to go gluten free makes the magnesium deficiency issue even worse because grains and cereals are some of the best sources of magnesium. So, when people cut these out, they are also cutting out lots of magnesium, which then further degrades the 300+ enzyme functions that require it–not all of those are digestive enzymes however. Like amino acids, your body can't and doesn't store magnesium; Therefore, you need to eat it every day in adequate amounts or you need to supplement it.

To give you some idea of just how important magnesium (Mg) is, consider these facts: every single living cell on Earth requires magnesium for life; every cell in your body is powered by the ATP (adenosine triphosphate) energy made in the mitochondria (power house of the cell), but the ATP is useless (biologically inactive) unless it is bound to a magnesium ion. What keeps every cell and you alive is really Mg-ATP. Briefly stated: no magnesium equals death.

There are worse effects though. Your DNA/RNA are dependant upon magnesium for their structure and function–you therefore can't have and make healthy cells that are "good replicas" without sufficient magnesium; Nor can your cells do their work to make proteins via messenger RNA. In terms of enzymes, the magnesium will at times bond to them and alter their structure so that they can even be able to do their work–they can contribute a water molecule that may be critical for that breaking up of the peptide glue/bond via hydrolysis; the magnesium is also a key part (a catalyst) of what allows the enzymes the right chemical environment/soup in which to work.

Bottom line: magnesium deficiency therefore means your enzymes can't work right. If your digestive enzymes can't work right, what hope do they have to completely break apart (or even to break apart what they can) the Superman alpha-gliadin-33-mer? Turned around, with sufficient magnesium, your enzymes have the tools they need to tackle Superman–magnesium is their kryptonite!

All of this is just the tip of the iceberg; I've read things about how magnesium is critical for literally thousands of the processes that go on in your body! Magnesium is so important to your body for so many functions that if you are deficient it leads to literally dozens of side effects and conditions: depression, chronic fatigue, weakness, dizziness, insomnia, calcium deficiency, poor heart health, muscle cramps, tremors, nausea, anxiety, high blood pressure, type II diabetes, respiratory issues, potassium deficiency, difficulty swallowing, poor memory, confusion, and on and on.

You can also find that magnesium deficiency leads to Irritable Bowel Syndrome; That is fascinating since we've already discussed its symptom list is about the same as gluten sensitivity and that it is also a gut related problem generally.

We can even put together several of the pieces of understand we already have to get a bigger picture of what is going on: certain foods hurt our villi and thus impair absorption of all nutrients; this means we can't absorb our magnesium enough or very well, and besides which most people don't even consume enough in the first place; magnesium deficiency then leads to our enzymes not working and also hurts the gut generally; we also need our probiotics/gut flora to help with digesting gluten, but taking antibiotics and/or candida overgrowth due to eating too much sugar and drinking too much alcohol can mostly wipe out our gut flora. The gut flora themselves require magnesium to live. This is a "perfect storm" or combination of things that puts our overall gut health in the toilet. Is it any wonder we have an issue digesting gluten with compromised and barely functioning gut/intestine, flora, and enzymes? So then we stop eating gluten and get even less magnesium. Further, if we don't do multiple things to repair our gut health (and stop or cut down on certain other foods), the cycle just continues even if we cut out gluten from our diet!

So, the big picture revelation is this: a number of contributing causes or culprits are occurring with gluten sensitivity/intolerance; each of these cascade, inter-relate, and affect each other; the overall combination creates the "perfect storm" of a very distressed and compromised gut that stands no chance of dealing with the Superman alpha-gliadin-33-mer. Addressing each of these, and doing some other things we will discuss, will "right the ship" and take us out of that "perfect storm" to calm waters and a calm gut.

So, I guess we should put getting enough magnesium on your list of things to do to "Fix Gluten Sensitivity and Heal Your Gut". Also, this will be true of everything I recommend doing to fix your gluten sensitivity: ensuring you are getting enough magnesium is a very good idea generally speaking and will improve many aspects of your health.

An interesting thought is that if one looks at how many magnesium deficient people there are and how many gluten sensitive people there are, then there is at least a correlation between them if not even possible causation. We will have to treat this as a possible theory as well. Even if magnesium deficiency isn't part of the cause, you have no hope of proper digestion and healthy enzymes without getting enough magnesium. So, even if it isn't causing the problem, it is likely at least contributing to it, and is most definitely a required part of any solution.

Before we finish up here, let's go back to the general idea that we likely have some problems with our gut health. Let's recall that leaky gut stuff and zonulin. Is it possible that this also compromises our gut flora? I mean this is the very place they call home and live inside. Even if this happens to be true, are there still other things that may have damaged our small intestine? We will explore that in the next chapter.

Bottom line key understandings are these: Gluten proteins and Gliadin in particular are just dang hard to digest even in the best of circumstances by a healthy person. In all likelihood the truth is that the human body cannot fully digest alpha-gliadin-33 without the help of bacteria/gut flora. It is therefore important to have a large and healthy colony of gut flora. To ensure our enzymes are doing the best job they can and to support our gut flora, it is also very important to ensure we are getting enough magnesium.

Chapter 7: Glyphosate as the Culprit?

We have gotten into a lot of details that actually helped reveal several things that are contributing to poor gut health and also why digesting gluten is just difficult in the best-case scenario. But, is there perhaps something else that is contributing and doing harm to our guts?

I still had an unshakable question even after I studied and research a ton about gliadin, how the small intestine works, and digestion of proteins. Recall my personal story from the beginning of this book. Also, I've heard many people say the exact same thing. Why is it that only recently did I develop a problem with gluten after eating it for decades?

I have a degree in Computer Science. I have done lots of computer software work in my life. I was trained to ask clients and myself this good question when some problem suddenly appeared seemingly out of nowhere: So, what has changed?

Logically I can deduce that only one of two things had changed: my body had changed; the wheat had changed. Now actually there is a third possibility that perhaps other foods had changed, my diet had changed, or something like I was exposed to environmental toxins in some form. However, I didn't consider that last possibility at the time due to my focus on the wheat creating the symptoms.

I considered the first option and thought there may be some merit and things to consider about my body changing. Firstly I have gotten older; It is either well known or widely believed that as we age we lose and/or have less digestive enzymes–consider older people eating lots of soup and very simple and bland foods. I could also over time have changes in my overall gut health via the multiple things we have already discussed: poor gut flora, damaged villi, magnesium deficiency, etc. So, we can keep these in mind and certainly put them in the category of "contributing factors/culprits".

Okay, so then I decided to tackle the only other logical thing that could have changed: the wheat itself. So, I dug into researching wheat, how it is grown, processed, hybridized, etc. In my research on the internet I included the keyword "change" to try to narrow down my results to hopefully uncover what had changed over my lifetime about the wheat. I also probably typed in something along the lines of, "What happened to wheat?"

It didn't take long to uncover an article and graph about wheat. These showed a strong correlation between a dramatic rise in Celiac disease over the same period of time as an increase in the use of glyphosate on wheat. Wheat is not a crop that has been genetically engineered (GE), or is a genetically modified organism (GMO). Note: there appears to be an approved GMO wheat, but like many approved crops it isn't being grown (yet). At any rate, this article had this graph and an explanation about the use of glyphosate/Roundup on wheat just prior to harvest. It also had information of studies showing glyphosate kills certain strains of our gut flora or probiotics. But the point is that it started me on the track of researching glyphosate.

We will delve deeply into what glyphosate is, but first we will start out very generally. Glyphosate is the main herbicide and chemical in the product Roundup made by the company Monsanto. Monsanto is also the company that makes the genetically engineered crops. For now, just understand that glyphosate kills nearly any plant. In order to use it on food crops, they (Monsanto) genetically engineered the crops to be able to withstand and live despite being exposed to glyphosate/Roundup. The question immediately arises, "Why would they use glyphosate on wheat crops if it is going to kill them because they aren't genetically engineered to withstand it?"

The simple and somewhat short answer is that wheat farmers use it in two ways or for two purposes: to ripen the wheat for better yield and to keep weeds out of the fields. The first way it is used is basically to intentionally kill the plant (and/or reduce its moisture content) at a specific/intentional time (as a desiccant). This is done to ensure it all ripens/dries and is ready to harvest at the same time in order to maximize yield. Otherwise it tends to ripen unevenly and there is no point in time where it is all perfectly ready at once.

So, glyphosate is being used to basically start the wheat's death process or dry it out because part of that natural cycle and process is to go to seed right before death at the end of the growing season to reproduce. This is done primarily in the more northern states/regions where the growing season is shorter and the types of wheat are different there as well. In the southern regions they are growing "winter wheat" (the majority of our wheat is of this type) and glyphosate isn't used in this way or for this purpose, but it is still used for the second purpose/reason.

The second reason it is used is to spray it on the land after harvest (or early the next year) to ensure the ground doesn't grow weeds the following season. Since weeds would otherwise come up in the early Spring, this means the farmer can plant sooner because they don't have to first spray those weeds and then wait a couple of weeks for them to die—or they get a jump start on this; Since glyphosate will kill the wheat, they can't wait until the crop is growing to fight the weeds using it. It is also done so that the field doesn't get taken over by weeds if/when they leave it unplanted for a year to recover (letting it lay fallow).

So, even though winter wheat doesn't get Roundup used as a desiccant, it still gets sprayed on the ground and it will leave some amount of residue. Roundup/glyphosate is also used as a desiccant on some oats and on oil seed rape crops. Oil seed rape is more commonly known as Canola and of course that gets used to make lots of Canola oil–which used to be a very healthy oil until they began this practice. Canola oil is commonly used for frying foods.

Even though wheat isn't GE/GMO, they still use glyphosate (Roundup) on it and the ground/fields it grows in.

Acting like a detective or sleuth, this article put me even more firmly on the trail of glyphosate. I realized I needed to investigate and study glyphosate since it seemed to be what had changed about the wheat. Sure enough, I found that they just started using it in 1990, its usage increased slowly over the years, and then it became more widespread and they have sprayed more and more of the stuff each year ever since. So this coincided with my working theory that something in the wheat had been changed and that is why I was able to eat it the previous decades of my life without issue–or so it seemed.

But I also found out in researching glyphosate generally that it was being used mainly for GMO crops such as corn, soy, sugar beets, and others. Later we will discuss in detail how just these few crops work their way into hundreds of foods we eat. So, maybe it wasn't just the wheat after all, maybe it was the glyphosate in general. Maybe that third logical category of what had changed was actually the answer: other foods/diet. This certainly would include the wheat, but this would mean it isn't necessarily that just eating the glyphosate-treated wheat is the problem, but that the problem is eating lots of glyphosate over time from a variety of food sources. Logically this would mean we could have a theory that the glyphosate trashes our gut and that this is simply most noticeable when we eat wheat due to how dang difficult it is to digest gliadin.

Therefore, we need to know the answer to this question: What is Glyphosate? Well, the National Pesticide Information Center (NPIC) "is a cooperative agreement between Oregon State University and the U.S. Environmental Protection Agency". As such, we might consider them basically "pro-glyphosate" or touting the company line. This is their short description of what it is: "Glyphosate is a non-selective herbicide, meaning it will kill most plants. It prevents the plants from making certain proteins that are needed for plant growth. Glyphosate stops a specific enzyme pathway, the shikimic acid pathway. The shikimic acid pathway is necessary for plants and some microorganisms."

Note the part at the end, "…and some microorganisms". One might wonder (and many have) if it affects the microorganisms called our gut flora or probiotics. We already have discussed this is a likely problem area related to an unhealthy gut and gliadin digestion. We will come back to this point shortly.

They go on to say, "…avoid exposure. If any exposures occur, be sure to follow the First Aid instructions on the product label carefully. For additional treatment advice, contact the Poison Control Center at 1-800-222-1222." So, if it isn't harmful and is as safe as they want us to think, why would all labels have warnings, First Aid instructions, etc?

The direction to contact poison control tells you clearly it is a toxic poison; it is only a matter of how much of this poison does what level of harm. There is a somewhat famous piece of video footage where an interview about glyphosate/roundup is being done with a Monsanto executive. The executive rambles on about how it is harmless to humans. Then the interviewer pushes a glass of glyphosate across the table to him and says something like, "What a relief. Since it is not harmful to humans, please drink this." Of course the guy didn't drink it.

NPIC goes on to state, "When high doses were administered to laboratory animals, some studies suggest that glyphosate has carcinogenic potential. Studies on cancer rates in people have provided conflicting results on whether the use of glyphosate containing products is associated with cancer. Some studies have associated glyphosate use with non-Hodgkin lymphoma. Glyphosate exposure has been linked to developmental and reproductive effects at high doses that were administered to rats repeatedly during pregnancy. These doses made the mother rats sick. The rat fetuses gained weight more slowly, and some fetuses had skeletal defects. These effects were not observed at lower doses."

This is sort of like they are saying, "Heck yes it is toxic and poisonous, but if you don't get too much then it isn't so bad." Feel better? Now keep in mind this organization is more likely to be minimizing glyphosate harms since they are working with the government's EPA who has approved the stuff and says it is safe for the environment and us. But, even they are admitting some unfavorable studies and issues with this poison. Other very biased and pro-glyphosate articles and sources say things like, "There are no reputable studies showing any harmful effects to humans (or causing cancer) from glyphosate."

One guy who was trying to debunk an article we will discuss later actually states that because humans don't have that shikimic acid pathway that plants do, glyphosate is safe for humans. Well, it may be true that it won't kill you in the same way as it kills plants. However, to suggest that a chemical isn't harmful to humans just because it hurts plants in a particular way is completely illogical. Technically this is called a "non-sequiter" argument, or it is saying, "this follows that" when there is actually no logical connection between the two points.

There is obviously the potential that it can be harmful to humans in perhaps multiple ways–a fact we will confirm later. In fact, that humans are different than plants actually means there may be many ways it damages us that were never intended or considered because they were focused on and looking only at the effects on the plants/weeds. Of course they tested and studied what it does to the weeds.

Did they study the effects of glyphosate and GMO food in long-term human trials to see if it did any harm or establish that it is safe? You would think they would be required to do that by something like the Food and Drug Administration (FDA)–like they have to do for new drugs. Actually they did not do any human trials, testing, studies, etc. In fact, they did just a few very short tests on rats; The longest of which was only two months. The "they" doing the testing was Monsanto themselves, and neither the FDA, EPA, nor anyone else did any testing at all prior to it being foisted upon the unsuspecting public.

How this is done reads like a movie script based upon a conspiracy theory–you might want to research it if you are interested. The short version is a guy was an attorney whose clients were Monsanto and another Biotech company. He wrote a paper for them, the government invented a new job/position for him, and once in that new position he edited the paper and the EPA/FDA adopted it as their position about GMO foods–how they say it is safe, fine, etc. The plot and apparent conspiracy gets better when this guy is known to have gone back and forth between working for the government and Monsanto itself directly. This type of arrangement and practice is called things like "the revolving door" or "the good old boys club". A recent director of the FDA was a former member of Monsanto's board of directors. Can you spell "conflict of interest", "conspiracy", or perhaps "corruption"?

Speaking of only doing short testing on rats, I smell a rat! In the end, they unleashed this stuff on the public without any clue, knowledge, testing, or data about what it would do to human bodies. In a way you are serving as the guinea pig or rat; Did you recall volunteering to test man-made chemicals and genetically engineered Frankenstein food? Heck, most of us hadn't even heard of

"Monsanto", "glyphosate", or "GMO foods" until after we had already been eating them for 10 to 20 years! Some people actually still haven't heard of them or don't know/understand much at all about them.

Well that is some short background and general information about glyphosate. But, since we got down into the details of Biochemistry on other matters, we better do the same for glyphosate and get a detailed definition and understanding of what this stuff really is:

Glyphosate is a glycine molecule with an additional methyl phosphonyl group attached to the nitrogen atom. Glycine is an amino acid! This means that basically glyphosate is a man-made, Frankenstein version of the glycine amino acid.

Some intelligent and knowledgeable people argue that a key mechanism of its "insidious cumulative toxicity" is its ability to substitute for glycine by mistake during protein synthesis. In other words, it is mostly all glycine and your body can get tricked into thinking it is normal/good glycine and using it as such–if so, big trouble ensues. Looking into the word parts of "glyphosate" we can see they chose that as a combination of the "gly" from glycine and the "phosate" part is related to the phosphonyl/phosphate.

Since it is this Frankenstein version of glycine and the body perhaps will accept/mistake it as such, we ought to know at least a little about glycine. Glycine is the simplest of all the 22 amino acids–it is like the smallest LEGO piece with just two prongs on top. As such, it can get used as a fundamental building block for making many types of proteins as our body reassembles amino acids. Interestingly, it works in concert with glutamine–recall that is our villi's spinach.

Glycine is the second most widespread amino acid found in human enzymes and proteins. Wait, did I just say "enzymes"? Yes, indeed. We will come back to this fact shortly. Glycine is also involved in the transmission of chemical signals in the brain and is considered by some to be a "brain booster". Since it helps make proteins, it is also a key component for making/building muscles, joint ligaments/tendons, bones, and forms a third of collagen.

Now then, it being a main ingredient of collagen is very important because glycine helps form two of the most important substances that make up the gut lining: collagen and gelatin. In fact, this is so well understood that supplementing glycine is often done to help people that have inflammatory bowel diseases (IBS), Crohn's disease, ulcerative colitis, and acid reflux. Additionally it is taken as a supplement to promote probiotics (gut flora) balance and growth because those require it as well. But there is much more to the story of this wonderful amino acid.

Within the intestinal tract, glycine also acts like a metabolic fuel. It's needed to manufacture bile, nucleic acids, creatine phosphate and porphyrins to be used to break down nutrients from your diet. In other words, it does many functions that are directly related to the entire digestive process happening properly. And remember that glycine is a key/major part of digestive enzymes as well.

But, what if your body somehow accepts glyphosate and thinks it is actually real/good glycine? Could it then make it's way into various parts of the body? Since it is different and also toxic, is it then going to have a cascading affect and impair these various systems? Remember how many of these are related to various parts and processes of the entire digestive tract?

What happens if your gut is trying to make digestive enzymes and uses glyphosate instead of glycine to do that? Do they not come out viable, are deformed, do not work at all, or just work poorly? Knowing how important the enzymes are, and that they already struggle with alpha-gliadin, this certainly could be an area for concern. Since glycine is used in combination with glutamine and our villi love glutamine, is glyphosate mistaken as glycine getting into our villi and killing them? Since our probiotics/gut flora use glycine, do they suffer the same fate(s)? What about the cells lining the gut that are collagen? Are new ones made with glyphosate that somehow makes them defective? If glycine is used in the bile system, could glyphosate get into our bile ducts? If so, might it fundamentally hurt them in some way? While we glossed over the digestive process where bile gets introduced, it is a necessary part.

They say glyphosate doesn't accumulate in our bodies and instead passes right thru us. By "they" I mean if you research what Monsanto, the governments (FDA/EPA), and the scientists promoting glyphosate or on the payroll say; Those talking heads are the "they" I mean. So they say it goes right in and out and therefore does no harm. That is apparently is not true according to multiple sources and testing.

Consider how this is either minimized or the discussion avoided by folks like NPIC, "The vast majority of glyphosate leaves the body in urine and feces without being changed into another chemical." Does that make you feel safe and better about it? The key words here are "vast majority". Also, who cares about "without being changed into another chemical" if it mimics glycine and if it is already a harmful chemical and poison in the first place?

But if you research elsewhere you find things like this turn up, "As Roundup producer Monsanto itself has reported, the residue from glyphosate tends to accumulate in the bones, marrow, and collagen-rich ligaments of animals. Dr. Anthony Samsel confirmed this finding in his own study of the bones, marrow, and other parts of pigs and cows, as well as the derived bovine gelatin." It should be noted that when he looked at vaccines that didn't use bovine/cow gelatin, there was no glyphosate residue. Dr. Samsel also looked at digestive enzymes such as trypsin and lipase. He found significant glyphosate residue in them. So we see right there it is getting inside and absorbed–at least in animals/cows. So, we may have discovered another answer to a previous question: Yes, it may very well be getting into our digestive enzymes as well.

Now the information from Dr. Samsel came from an article that was focusing on cancer, autism, and other diseases being linked to the MMR vaccine, which is known to contain glyphosate. It has glyphosate residue/contamination because those animal tissues are used in the culture medium to grow the viruses contained in vaccines and because it is also in the gelatin used as a stabilizer in vaccines. It has the glyphosate as a contaminant because the animal tissues contain it. Of course they got it because they (cows) were fed GMO corn with glyphosate used on it and with residue of it getting into the corn kernels. We like to test things on rats and animals because they are actually quite similar to humans for most biological functions; Therefore if it is known that glyphosate ends up in all those types of animal tissues then we can logically induce it is highly likely that ends up in ours as well.

Since it is known multiple animal tissues contain glyphosate, it is highly likely that glyphosate bio-accumulates in our tissues and bodies! If true, this means it does NOT just pass right thru us with no harm done.

The detailed Biochemistry of how glyphosate ends up inside tissues, etc. is perhaps too complex for our purposes. However, a very brief overview gives us a look at how it might be that glyphosate gets embedded within the human body–contrary to the claims and assurances often cited that it doesn't do this and "passes right through us". There are 8 enzymes (or tissues) called transglutaminase in our bodies; They are also found in plants. Basically they are involved in building up complex and strong proteins by assembling amino acids. So, this isn't related to digestion and breaking things apart, but how things are constructed and then used within the human body or plants.

When these enzymes go to work, people with Celiac disease then generate anti-transglutaminase antibodies, which may play a role in the small bowel damage in response to dietary gliadin. Therefore, there seems to be something about these processes whereby glyphosate does get incorporated into things that can end up as part of tissues, enzymes, etc. Since plants also use transglutaminase, this likely means the plant cells themselves get embedded with glyphosate by using transglutaminase enzymes. In other words, it gets inside the food itself.

The bottom line points are these: it is highly likely that glyphosate is not just like some dust or residue that doesn't get inside the food itself, or that can be washed off–it is very likely that it actually becomes a part of what we eat; If true, glyphosate would then likewise become a part of the human body due to being mistaken for glycine and utilized by transglutaminase to make proteins, which are then used and embedded in certain cells, tissues, enzymes, etc.

The article is by Dr. Stephanie Seneff, who has done a number of articles that are basically sounding alarms about glyphosate. Her articles and others in a similar vein are also raising some ruckus and pushback by those who support GMO foods and the use of glyphosate. Some of her critics were quick to mention that she is a senior scientist at MIT and Computer Science is her expertise. However, they omit the facts that she has an undergraduate degree in Biology from MIT, and a minor in food and nutrition. She also works with some large organizations and colleagues directly in the related fields. I think that means she is fairly qualified, and certainly not totally unqualified on the subject. What they are attempting to do here is a form of "character assassination" or in logic it is known as the fallacy of an "ad hominem". In Latin that means "to the person" and it is used as a tactic of attacking the person themselves instead of what they are saying/claiming–usually due to having no factual or valid way to refute the claims themselves.

Most of this next part she said could likely be found in a Biology textbook. Perhaps she is just putting two and two together, or maybe she availed herself of her colleagues or other studies/sources to reach this revealing statement: "The cells that form these villi, called enterocytes, begin life as an undifferentiated stem cell in the 'crypt' area of the intestines. From there, they proliferate and mature as they migrate up the walls of the crypt, and then settle in on the surface of the villi, where they absorb nutrients before dying and getting replaced by new arrivals in a constant renewal process. Glyphosate, as an amino acid, is actively imported into cells along L-type amino acid transporters. Cells that proliferate, like enterocytes, express high levels of these transporters, and therefore preferentially take up glyphosate."

The simplified bottom line is that your gut villi sort of love and soak up glyphosate! So, just a moment ago I had asked if it could get mistaken for glycine and taken into the body. We know glycine is the simplest amino acid and makes up muscles, collagen, bones, digestive enzymes, etc. We know when they use/study these tissues from animals, and even enzymes from people, they do indeed find glyphosate in them. Therefore the answer seems to be this:

Yes, it is very likely that glyphosate gets mistaken for glycine and may be stored/used where glycine is used–including our all-important villi, and/or that transglutaminase tissues and enzymes utilize it. We have absolutely found glyphosate inside many types of animal tissues. Our same tissues are made in the same ways, and from the same chemicals and processes. Like plants, we also use transglutaminase. Therefore, it is quite logical and highly probable that glyphosate does the same thing in humans–accumulates inside our bodies at the cellular level.

This would mean that glyphosate is getting into our gut lining itself, villi, enzymes, and many other places. In fact, a good question might be, "Just where in our bodies does glyphosate not go, wreak havoc, and accumulate?" As a small side note: this is another possible way or reason that glyphosate basically becomes stuck, lodged, or embedded in the small intestine's walls (the collagen tissue).

If this glyphosate is being taken in as mistaken glycine and accumulating in our bodies, we can see multiple major issues this is causing due to all the places and ways glycine is utilized. Most directly to our topic, it is going to mess up several important things: the collagen/lining of our small intestine, our villi, our colony of gut flora, our digestive enzymes, and our bile and other things elsewhere in our digestive tract.

The main point I'm making is that glyphosate probably accumulates and/or get used in the body. This would be the amount that is not part of the "vast majority" NPIC tried to gloss over. Based upon their omissions and double-speak already noted, I'm not sure I even believe this "vast majority" claim. In fact, when you read most any "pro-glyphosate" talking-head or paid shill, you will almost always find this same sort of statement as that repeated, "Glyphosate doesn't accumulate and just passes right through us without doing any harm." Now we have multiple reasons and evidence that suggest this is very likely to be false. Any article stating things like that would appear to be biased and attempting to minimize or flat-out cover-up the harms of glyphosate. Accordingly, if you do independent research and find such statements, you can strongly consider the possibility that they are bogus, biased, and deceptive.

In researching glyphosate I also uncovered another fascinating fact that, when explored and considered, reveals another entire way glyphosate is compromising our body. Glyphosate was first patented as a pipe cleaner due to its remarkable ability to chelate metals–this wasn't a Monsanto patent, but a patent by Stauffer Chemical in 1964. "Chelation" is a process of metals getting stuck to a carrier via hydrogen bonding.

Just think of chelation as the base material having a magnetic gluey surface that attracts and attaches nearby metals to it. In terms of our bodies, this "chelation" means that glyphosate chemically bonds to metals and takes them out of the bloodstream, or out of our "slurry/soup" of nutrients in the small intestine. So, this means the "vast majority" (or whatever portion) that does exit our system is then carrying away a bunch of metals along with it.

We may not normally think of metals as being vital nutrients, but they certainly are. They are typically categorized as "minerals", but minerals also include things like salts, sulfur, phosphorus, chlorine, etc. There are also a fair number of these important metal minerals: copper, zinc, iron, manganese, etc. Do you remember our old friend magnesium that we talked so much about and the many things we need it for? Yep, you guessed it…magnesium is an alkaline Earth metal!

Recall that every living cell needs magnesium, and how one gut flora needs manganese (among other minerals and metals like magnesium). When we see how glyphosate is bonding with these metals and taking them out of our system, we see it is hijacking, robbing, and making a getaway with some precious resources that our probiotics/gut flora require to live. Of course our villi, collagen/lining need these same things as well. Would you suppose that things like our enzymes or hormones might also require these essential minerals including the metals? Indeed they do. So once again this is a way our gut gets negatively impacted because our digestive enzymes need these metals that glyphosate is stealing. It is like a thief stealing our gold and silver–our precious metals.

The bottom line: Glyphosate bonds to (chelates) vital nutrient metals and takes them out of our blood and small intestine's digested food stuffs. Without these, our gut flora die off and the health of our villi are compromised. Without these our ability to make hormones and digestive enzymes is limited. Since we already know that villi, enzymes, hormones, and gut flora are all essential to digesting and absorbing gliadin and many other nutrients, glyphosate is compromising our gut health in multiple ways that degrade our ability to fully digest gluten/gliadin in addition to other foods. Since these same metals are critically important to literally hundreds of our body's functions, there are also an untold number of other negative consequences to our health.

The important point is that glyphosate is basically robbing your body of multiple critically important metal nutrients such as iron, manganese, and magnesium. Most people already aren't getting enough of these–in particular magnesium. This means glyphosate is depriving us of what little we do eat. So glyphosate is compromising our gut health indirectly since magnesium is critical to gut flora, the small intestine walls, digestive enzymes, and villi. When our gut health is compromised it leads to a downward spiral: our gut and digestive system is no longer able to fully absorb nutrients, but these are the very same nutrients it requires to repair itself. Put another way, glyphosate trashes your gut in numerous ways and then adds insult to injury by injecting itself into repairs being made at the cellular level (mistaken as glycine) and also by stealing away key metals that all parts of the system need in order to be repaired and maintain health. Our gut gets messed up and can't repair itself because it is messed up, which in turn makes it weaker and more vulnerable to getting even worse. If we get into this cycle and keep dumping in glyphosate, then this downward spiral continues.

Let's get back to Dr. Stephanie Seneff who had written the article with the graph showing Celiac/glyphosate correlation and talking about glyphosate usage on wheat. The graph shows the sharp rise of the use of glyphosate/Roundup on wheat over the past two decades, which is also overlaid with a nearly identical sharp rise in Celiac disease.

The article and graph generated a fairly big stir and were circulated, referenced, and re-published fairly widely. Ever since then there have been people attacking the author as well as how it inaccurately over-focused on glyphosate being widely used as a desiccant on wheat–whereas in truth the majority of it is used for the next year's weed control on winter wheat. If you assume those attacking the article and data might have a vested interest in promoting Roundup and trying to reassure the public it is safe, then you are making a pretty wise assumption.

The graph and article I read was very damning and appear to show very strong correlation between the increased usage of glyphosate/Roundup on wheat and Celiacs disease. What is particularly strange about this are two things. Here is the first one: Celiac is supposedly genetic; the graph shows "new incidence" or diagnosis rates; now then, if it is a genetic disease, how could it have surged from about 20,000 a year to 80,000 a year between 1992 and

2010? This could only have happened if for some reason people with Celiacs spontaneously started having 9 children a year instead of the average 2.3 or so. This makes no sense whatsoever.

The second strange thing is that this graph shows a stronger/tighter correlation than if you compared Celiacs to other GMO crops such as corn or soy. In other words, it is a near perfect match–including a little downturn/decrease at exactly the same time for Celiacs and glyphosate usage amounts on wheat. However, it is also still strongly correlated to the rate/graph of the use of glyphosate generally, which ties into the theory that glyphosate from any food source is the real issue–it isn't just from the wheat, but the gliadin in the wheat creates the major and most notable symptoms.

People that tried to de-bunk the graph and article like to throw out that "correlation does not equal causation", which is true. Sometimes it does, but sometimes it doesn't. So, just because two things are similar does not mean that one definitely causes the other. For example, you could do a study and then make a graph that shows that 95% of people that suffer heart attacks also had automatic-drip coffee makers in their home. But, this does not mean that coffee makers cause heart attacks. It also does not mean that having a heart attack magically makes a coffee maker appear in your kitchen.

Unfortunately for the pro-glyphosate shills and hucksters trying to debunk the data, the original source of the graph (Nancy L. Swanson), produced many other graphs on a wide variety of illnesses and diseases. They all show pretty much the same thing: when you graph the various diseases right on top of the use of glyphosate (or in some cases volume of GMO crops), you see they match nearly perfectly. Swanson also did legitimate statistical analysis to try to see if the correlation was indeed pointing to causation. She utilized a common statistical formula that uses the Pearson's correlation coefficient to determine how closely correlated the two data sets are. A standard interpretation of it says that if the coefficient **"r" = +.70 or higher**, then there is a *"very strong positive relationship."*

All of the graphs/data analyzed scored higher than .92 and this includes these: Thyroid Cancer, Liver Cancer, Obesity, Diabetes, Autism, Alzheimer's (deaths), Parkinson's (deaths), Dementia (deaths). Just to give you an idea how damning these statistical analyses are, consider that even an r value from +.40 to +.69 is considered a "strong positive relationship". So these values sort of scream "Oh heck yes we have an issue/cause and direct relationship between these diseases and glyphosate/GMO crops!"

These graphs and tables of data they are based upon show the trends/increase of the diseases from 1990 to 2010 because glyphosate first came into use in 1990 and the research was done in 2013 and the disease data was only available up until 2010. Now a de-bunker may claim these diseases were on the rise before glyphosate entered the picture. However, they would be wrong and she also covered her bases on that front. She prepared graphs that include the disease/condition data/rates for the 10 years prior and you can see they are either flat or on very slow increasing trends. This allows you to see where they "would have been" but for the glyphosate, GMO crops, and pesticide usage.

It's important to understand that these are radical rates of increase. We see things like 14 times the number of deaths by intestinal infection, 4 times more inflammatory bowel disease, and 10 times the number of deaths from dementia. I could go on and on, but the numbers are all similar and you should check it out for yourself. I will mention just three more specifically.

The number of children with diagnosed with autism each year went from about 1,500 to 37,000!!! (Note those are guesstimates based on a hard to read graph due to its scale). I and many people hadn't even heard of autism 25 years ago and it was certainly incredibly rare; Now it seems everyone is talking about it, knows about it, and it has become common. On an easier to read graph we can see the chances of your child being born with autism used to be about 1 in 5,000 back in 1990, but that skyrocketed to about 1 in 100 in 2010. I just saw another source give about the same historic data and that now in 2017 it is up to 1 in 36!!!

Why this incredible surge in autism? Some say it is from the vaccinations–mostly this is thought to be related to the mercury and other toxic metals, but we already know that these vaccines actually contain glyphosate as well! It is very likely a combination of the metals, other toxins, and glyphosate–the vaccines are a basically a toxic cocktail. Beyond that, kids nowadays are bombarded by glyphosate in most every food and drink they consume. Perhaps mistaken for glycine or glutamine, it acts like glutamine and goes right to the brain.

This same skyrocketing rate is true of diabetes. In the years between 1980 and 1991 the new incidents are so low they don't even appear on the graph and I'm just guessing on the tiny ones that do appear it may have been about 5,000 to 10,000, but less than 5,000 for multiple years. The rate of increase tracks precisely along the path of the graph showing the increase usage of glyphosate and ends with a rate about 1.1 million per year. So from less than 5,000 to over a million! Wow!

When I was growing up and even into mid-life, I'd never heard of ADHD. Had you? I'm not even sure if they had that label for it yet or perhaps it never even existed until recently. Well of course now tons of kids have it and they put them on drugs like Ritalin to try to control it. Great, drug the kids for what likely relates to diet and could therefore be fixed by diet. So ADHD is on this same sharp rise and tracks with GMO foods and glyphosate usage increases. What might be the connection?

More relevant to our topic, Swanson has graphs, data, and studies related to our guts and various ailments: bile duct cancer, intestinal infection, function bowel disorder, irritable bowel, constipation, peritonitis (perforated of part of the GI tract), inflammatory bowel disease, Crohn's disease, ulcerative colitis, and of course "leaky gut". All of these graphs show the exact same trends matching nearly perfectly with glyphosate/GMO trends. Based upon these statistics, it certainly seems obvious that the GMO food and glyphosate is wiping out our guts!

After you see all of these graphs and read up on the specific mechanisms about how glyphosate causes disruptions and does damage, it sure seems rather obvious the stuff is literally rotting our guts out, trashing our overall gut health, and this then leads to multiple effects and consequences. It becomes pretty obvious to a reasonable person that glyphosate is the main culprit and that just one of many consequences is gluten sensitivity. While we may not yet be able to prove with 100% certainty all this is occurring, it seems way more likely than not.

So, an investigation into what has changed about wheat led me to an article and graph about glyphosate usage. I then delved into the details of glyphosate and what the heck it is and does, which we have mostly already covered. Like a detective, I was simply following the leads I encountered and chasing them down to "get the facts and get to the bottom of this mystery."

I wanted to include the graph from the original article I found a couple of years ago in my initial research. Since I don't have permissions to use it, I'm not going to include it. Besides that, in trying to find a quality copy I traced the graph's origin to Nancy L. Swanson. So that is how I just got a lot of the information we just covered.

In 2013 there was a potential ballot issue to vote on GMO food labels in Washington state. Swanson published a series of articles in the Seattle examiner in an obvious attempt to increase public awareness of just how horrible these things are to our health. I highly recommend you read the 42-page document that was the content of the full published series, **"Genetically Modified Organisms and the deterioration of health in the United States" by Nancy L. Swanson.**

At a minimum you might want to at least skim it and view all of the graphs–a picture is worth a thousand words. If you do read it, you will find a lot more details about just how many areas of your body are trashed by glyphosate, just how many conditions and illnesses are either caused or made much worse by it, and have some proof, evidence, data, and a bunch of links and citations to numerous other studies in support of this position. In other words, after reading it I think you will be sufficiently convinced; Beyond being relevant to gluten sensitivity, it will open your eyes to many much worse things that will likely happen to you and your loved ones if you keep eating their Frankenstein GMO food–Frankenfood and consuming glyphosate. It certainly had that affect on me, and it was a great source for further evidence and confirmation of the theory I had already arrive at: It's the glyphosate!

In my earlier research and ongoing research I've found tons of evidence, studies, and biochemical reasons glyphosate is really nasty stuff that does a lot of harm and damage. One could write a long book just about that topic and indeed many have done so. So, I can't cover all of that. But let me at least perhaps save you some time and also give the highlights and important things so you have more knowledge about it. If you are the more skeptical type of reader or really want to dig into and know the details, then by all means do your own research.

I want to begin by discussing hormones a little. Hormones were previously mentioned briefly in terms of requiring the magnesium that glyphosate steals. Also, they use/need glycine to be made and function and we know that glyphosate gets mistaken for it due to being a Frankenstein version of glycine. The importance of this is that your hormones control and regulate nearly every process in your body. They signal things to turn on, to turn off, to stay at certain levels, etc. If and when your hormones get messed up, lots of things in-turn go haywire. One example is that a key place that makes and releases hormones is the thyroid. It turns out that studies show glyphosate has the capacity to disrupt thyroid hormone functions, which is the primary issue with ADHD–now we might know the connection to that condition.

In terms of digestion, hormones regulate and control nearly every part of the process beginning by using hormones that make us feel hungry and get us to eat in the first place. A hormone gastrin triggers release of the stomach acids, hormones order the release of bile, and hormones are what get the gall bladder, pancreas, and small intestine to do their jobs. Hormones even communicate the orders about what to build from the nutrients and where to send things. Based upon this, you can see that if hormones get disrupted then so does our digestive process and systems all along the gastro-intestinal tract.

However, the hormone story gets even worse because there are also lots of cells in your gut that do work there making hormones that go to other system/places as well–for example making neurotransmitters that the brain needs. These specialized hormone-making cells are called enteroendocrine cells. In your GI tract they produce hormones such as serotonin, somatostatin, motilin, cholecystokinin, gastric inhibitory peptide, neurotensin, vasoactive intestinal peptide, and enteroglucagon. So if glyphosate is generally damaging the GI tract and messing up the environment, then these cells aren't going to be able to do their job right and make the required hormones. So, glyphosate has been shown by some to be a "hormone disruptor"; Its presence in our GI tract is going to mess with our hormones that in turn do tons of jobs in many areas of the body.

For example, that serotonin goes to your brain and makes you feel good; If that gets disrupted, then depression is a natural result; Recall that depression is a symptom of gluten sensitivity. You see, this suggests it isn't the gluten that makes you depressed, it is glyphosate disrupting your hormones combined with your generally ill gut damaged by glyphosate regardless of having eaten gluten–since glyphosate comes from many crops and sources.

Not only does glyphosate seem to mess with our hormones (endocrine system) in the two major ways already mentioned, but also there is another character in the GMO story that messes up our hormones and hormonal/endocrine system. It is a long story and outside the scope of our book, but the short version is that along with modifying crops to withstand glyphosate, many crops are also genetically modified to include something that kills pests as well: Bt toxin. It has enough bearing and relation to our topic that it is worth going into it somewhat briefly.

What they do is to take these bacteria they know kills pests, Bacillus thuringiensis (Bt), and shove a part of its DNA into the plant cells of the crop. They then grow a new plant from this and end up with seeds that will have these Bt toxic bacteria in them. When insects eat this stuff it does this: "…the toxin binds to receptors in the insect's gut, causing the gut wall to break down and allowing toxin spores and normal gut bacteria to enter the body. As spores and bacteria proliferate in the body, the insect dies." Doesn't this sound eerily similar? Sounds exactly like what we have been discussing about the break down of the intestinal wall and then "leaky gut".

How about just for fun we re-read that and change "insect" to "human"–and modify the end slightly. "When the Bt toxin in GMO crops is eaten by humans, the toxin binds to receptors in our gut, causing the gut wall to break down and allowing toxin spores and normal gut bacteria to enter the human body. As spores and bacteria proliferate in the body, the person will manifest many illnesses and then eventually dies." Could this happen to humans? Is this Bt toxin in GMO food harmful to us? Keep in mind "they" told us glyphosate is safe and doesn't hurt us, but now we know better than to simply take their word for that–and hopefully not to take their word for other questionable things.

Again, it is a long story but our infamous "they" will say this doesn't happen to humans and they quote studies about putting the Bt toxin in simulations of the gut, or testing it on rats. Both of these will show it doesn't cause harm. However, you can dig deeper and find another study that confirms those same findings, but adds a twist to the findings. In that study, when they gave the Bt toxin in straight form to the rats it actually didn't harm them, but when they fed the rats potatoes that had the Bt toxin embedded in it, it had several noticeable and damaging effects to the rats and their offspring. What is even more profound about this second study (done by Russian scientists I believe) is that the amount of Bt toxin in the potatoes was tiny compared to the direct Bt that was fed directly, which was 800 times the amount. This means that even very tine/trace amounts can do damage when embedded within food.

In other words, this study suggests/shows that it is the combination of the Bt toxin itself along with being embedded in the proteins/carbs that causes the problem and damage! Of course that combo and embedding in the cells themselves is exactly the GMO food we eat! So, this study's findings suggest that all the tests where Bt was given in isolated form do not tell the full and accurate story and are fundamentally flawed; In fact, they mislead one to believe the Bt toxins are harmless when they clearly are not. If you research Bt you will find that these likely flawed studies are quoted and referenced as proof that Bt toxins are safe. For example, look it up in Wikipedia and you will see this exact type of flawed testing as their only basis for saying it doesn't harm people. They even discuss how they gave huge amounts to rats and it did no harm and then point out those amounts are much greater than what we are taking in; But of course we know from the Russian study that this actually proves nothing at all and that small amounts actually do harm when they are inside the food itself.

As a side note, the Russians have decided to ban and not allow GMO foods or glyphosate in their country. Certainly they studied it prior to making this decision. As we already know, it was not studied in humans or even thoroughly tested in rats in the United States. So, who is more likely to know the truth on the matter? The Russians studied microwave ovens long ago and found they kill off all the vitamins; They banned microwaves for over 25 years in their country. Regardless of what you might think about the Russians, it would appear they have a genuine concern for the health of their people.

Another study at the University of Brasilia found that even in very low does it led to microcytic hypochromic anemia in mice–basically is trashed the cell walls of red blood cells and led to a big drop in red blood cell counts. Keep in mind this was just the pure toxin they tested. It seems highly unlikely based upon these studies and others that the Bt toxin is harmless to humans–particularly when it is inside the cells of the plants we eat.

The bottom line is that Bt toxins in GMO food are another potential culprit and issue. In addition to their gut rotting potential, there is another horrible thing about them. They are known by some to be hormone disruptors. In other words, it blocks your hormones from being able to do their many jobs–including all the ones related to digestion. It was because we just discussed the importance of hormones that I wanted to throw just a little information your way about this other villainous character in the tragic drama of GMO foods. Bt toxins may be like the evil twin brother of glyphosate. The two together do a one-two punch to the gut and also to hormone function!

That said, my personal opinion is that glyphosate does more harm in more ways. Another reason to mention the Bt toxin is because it may do some things glyphosate does not; It may be the primary cause of the sharp rise in certain bowel infections, leaky gut, Crohn's, etc. But, based upon what you now know about glyphosate, it sure seems to be acting as a secondary cause or contributing factor. However, the Bt toxins and glyphosate most often go hand-in-hand because they have crops, like corn, that are "stacked" to include both the genetic engineering for the herbicide Roundup AND the Bt toxin as a pesticide. The point is that if you are eating GMO foods then you are getting a lot of both of these likely evil twins.

Let's now move on to a summary of the highlight of other things my research turned up about glyphosate. I am not making these claims/statements personally, but only giving a survey of what others have claimed and found evidence to support: Glyphosate/Roundup makes worse and compounds the effects of other chemicals and toxic residues in our food supply; It stimulates hormone-dependant cancers even at very small levels; While we lack that shikimic/shikimate pathway that glyphosate uses to kill plants, bacteria do have it and that is why it kills our probiotics/gut flora; It disrupts your body making aromatic amino acids [likely due to the glycine confusion we discussed] which leads to amino acid deficiencies; It causes impairment of sulfate transport and sulfur metabolism leading to sulfate deficiency [this is the likely cause of the sharp rise in multiple sclerosis as this primarily affects the brain and a Dr. that cured herself of it focused on getting more sulfur]; It creates ammonia as a byproduct when microbes break down glyphosate, which can lead to brain inflammation associated with autism and Alzheimer's disease; It promotes aluminum accumulation in the brain–huge issue/cause of autism and perhaps Alzheimer's as well; It leads to nutritional deficiencies–especially minerals–and systemic toxicity [which normally your gut flora help eliminate for you]; It can disrupt the Vitamin A (retinoic acid) signaling pathway, which is crucial for normal fetal development; It messes up estrogen (female hormone) receptors, which leads to breast cancer; reduces testosterone (male hormone) levels, which contributes to diabetes; It can induce severe tryptophan deficiency, which can lead to an extreme inflammatory bowel disease [tryptophan is also the building block of serotonin and nearly every brain neurotransmitter–recall the "foggy brain" symptom and depression]; It disrupts liver cell function; It can induce the cell death that causes Parkinson's disease; It is toxic to human placental cells; It induces a shift in gut bacteria towards endotoxin-producing bacteria strongly associated with obesity.

I could go on and on with this list and you are free (and encouraged) to do your own research until you are sufficiently convinced this is nasty stuff. But based upon my research, instead of asking "In what ways does glyphosate harm our health, and what biological systems and processes does it affect?" it seems to me the better question with a much shorter answer is, "In what ways does glyphosate NOT harm our health, and what biological systems and processes are NOT negatively affected by it?"

In view of all this and if these things are true, then you might consider that if you only have gluten intolerance going on, then you are quite lucky for now; But, if you don't get off the GMO Frankenfood and glyphosate, then an entire host of other chronic illnesses, conditions, and diseases is looming on the horizon you are sailing towards.

There is so much mounting evidence about this that the Academy of Environmental Medicine has issued a position statement on GMO food stating, "...several animal studies indicate serious health risks associated with GM food consumption including infertility, immune dysregulation, accelerated aging, dysregulation of genes associated with cholesterol synthesis, insulin regulation, cell signaling, and protein formation, and changes in the liver, kidney, spleen and gastrointestinal system…There is more than a casual association between GM foods and adverse health effects. There is causation as defined by Hill's Criteria in the areas of strength of association, consistency, specificity, biological gradient, and biological plausibility. The strength of association and consistency between GM foods and disease is confirmed in several animal studies." They further state that "because GM foods have not been properly tested for human consumption, and because there is ample evidence of probable harm, we call on physicians to educate the public and warn their patients to avoid GM/GMO foods."

You see, everyone wants to be carefully about stating flat out that these things cause harm due to the potential for a lawsuit; Note their language and caveat of sorts, "…probable harm".

In fact, the radical rise in those many conditions and diseases we discussed can all be added together. When that is done a mind-blowing and heart-wrenching statistic comes out: 25% (or 1 in 4) of adults in the United States now suffer from **multiple** chronic diseases. This has basically double in 20 years. But, consider that while GMO foods began hitting the market in 1990, there was a slow increase and it is only the past 10 years where the amount of it has been substantial. For children in the United States, the chronic disease rate has increased from 12.8% in 1994 to 26.6% in 2006–It is even worse now, as we are 12 years beyond that statistic.

Let's shift gears slightly and put a nail in the coffin. Remember how Monsanto only did some short-term rat tests and the longest was a mere 2 months? You might wonder what would happen if the rats had been fed GMO food their entire lives. Well, you don't have to wonder because finally in 2012 a study was published that did just that.

This study found that rats fed a type of GM corn that is prevalent in the US food supply for two years developed massive mammary tumors, kidney, and liver damage, and other serious health problems. In females, all treated groups died 2-3 times more than controls, and more rapidly. Females developed large mammary tumors almost always more often than and before controls; The pituitary was the second most disabled organ. In treated males, liver congestions and necrosis were 2.5-5.5 times higher. Marked and severe kidney nephropathies were also generally 1.3-2.3 greater. Males presented 4 times more large palpable tumors than controls, which occurred up to 600 days earlier than in the controls. Biochemistry data confirmed very significant kidney chronic deficiencies; for all treatments and both sexes, 76% of the altered parameters were kidney related. These results can be explained by the non-linear endocrine-disrupting [hormone-disrupting] effects of Roundup, but also by the over-expression of the transgene in the GMO and its metabolic consequences.

One has to wonder if this study–and countless similar ones–had been done and reported to the FDA prior to GMO/Roundup being used in the U.S. if they would have approved it. In fact, it seems that all of the tests and studies done have been more than a decade "after-the-fact"; It seems only after serious consequences were already appearing did real science get done. It sure would have been nice to have the research and data before using humans in the U.S. and worldwide as rats and guinea pigs.

Imagine if you were approached to participate in a human trial of this Frankenfood, but they first gave you an information package for legal reasons and asked you to sign a waiver holding them harmless for anything that happened to you. Imagine that in this package it contained a dozen studies showing it caused multiple horrible side-affects, diseases, and even premature death. After looking through it all, would you have volunteered? Would you have signed the waiver? Even if they offered to pay you to be in the trial, would you have done it? How much money would be enough that you would risk your health and life? Ironically and tragically, you weren't even given the information package, research, and didn't knowingly consent to participate in the trial; It just sort of snuck into your food supply and most all of us ate it without even knowing it was in there–or at best knowing very little about it.

In fact, we couldn't know much about GMO food and glyphosate even if we had tried to educate ourselves before eating it because there simply was no significant and good research, studies, trials, or good science we could have used to make an informed and intelligent choice. Well, now we do have quite a bit of that, and likely a sufficient amount. Now you do know to some degree what this Frankenfood and toxic Glyphosate/Roundup chemical is very probably doing to your body. So, the question becomes this: Now that you know, are you still going to participate in this human trial?

I've mentioned a few times that if/when you research this topic you will find conflicting information or opinions. Generally speaking, one source is from some "camp" that is pro-GMO due to being hired and paid by Monsanto or other biotech companies, or working for some group that is somehow connected to them or the industry. If you dig a bit, you will even find stories of scientists hired to do testing and studies that did good science and produced results and conclusions showing it was harmful; Their findings were not used and they were fired–some of them even "black-listed" and couldn't find employment afterwards. There are stories you can find about scientists being hired and basically told ahead of time, "This is what we want you to show/prove: that it is safe/harmless." Well, scientists are not supposed to start with the conclusion, but are supposed to discover it based upon the experiments, studies, tests, science and evidence those produce.

Even the initial studies and tests on rats done by Monsanto were obviously flawed due to the short duration; The Bt studies didn't test the Bt toxin embedded in food. Worse, the testing being done by the company that makes the product and stands to make billions from it seems an obviously flawed practice that is way too open to the possibilities of bias, inadequacy, omission of certain findings, minimization, statistical manipulation, or even downright fraud. They have zero incentive to show negative impact and 100% incentive to show it is harmless and fine.

Let's say you wanted to find out the health benefits or dangers of some supplement, super food, herb, or health product. You do a search on the internet by entering its name. Now let's say 50 results and articles come up from university studies, online Biochemistry textbooks, non-profit organizations related to health, etc. But, you also get search results for 10 websites that are selling this stuff. Which of these two general types of results are you going to read in order to get the actual facts? Certainly you want the unbiased truth.

Of course the 10 websites are going to all say how wonderful and effective it is. Some of the other 50 pages may say it is beneficial, but many may say it does nothing valuable or even point out some risks, harms, etc. You don't seriously think the people/websites selling the stuff are going to put out that it "does nothing", can do harm, or has risks do you? In short, it is unwise and illogical to try to get the truth of a matter by using and relying upon the claims made by the producer or seller of a product–it is beyond doubt that they are biased and will only present positive information (and perhaps even exaggerated or false claims).

The point is to keep these things in mind if/when you do your own research. Also, you want to watch out for something called "confirmation bias", which is when you unconsciously seek out only the information that supports the belief or position you already have in mind. This happens easily in doing internet research just by how you choose the words of your search terms. For example (and I'm making no comment or opinion about vaccines), if you have heard or believe vaccines are harmful, then you might type in "Harmful effects of vaccines". You will get tons of results and they will all discuss the many harms, issues, etc. If you go study all of those search results and articles for two weeks, you will likely become convinced they are harmful–you will have confirmed the bias you started out with.

But, what if you had initially typed, "Benefits safety harm danger vaccines" into a search engine? You would have found a variety of results, studies, articles, etc. that would have been "on both sides of the issue". You can then study them all and make up your own mind as best you could. Alternatively, you could have done that first search and then done another one and typed in "benefits and safety of vaccines" to get the other side.

Unfortunately, for most any controversial subject you can find what seems compelling cases made for both sides. A couple of things we can do are to use our brains and wisdom where possible. We can "consider the source": who is saying this; who is paying/funding this person or organization that benefits financially from this position?

For example, you can see how considering the source of the FDA/EPA position and position paper on GE/GMO food would have led to revealing the bias, crony capitalism, good old boys club, and revolving door we already discussed. Knowing this, you can then pretty much know it is all going to be biased, bogus, incorrect, manipulated, and untrustworthy. Note: there are claims and even a lawsuit about how the FDA scientists that had warned about the dangers of GMO food were silenced and their research covered up–FDA documents appearing to prove this have been released.

Another example would be if you saw a headline and article on social media that said, "Scientists determine oil fracking doesn't pollute groundwater!" So then you research the author's name and find out he is employed directly by a fracking company; Or you find out he works for a research company, then check them out, and find out they have a contract with the fracking company. Is this a trustworthy source you think you are going to get the truth and unbiased facts from? But, what if you do this same research and find out it was based on a compilation of studies conducted by 7 universities and 25 different cities and counties across the country? That might engender a bit more trust in the content. You would still be wise to search for research, studies, and articles that perhaps showed ground water pollution near fracking.

As I've done my research I've tried to watch out for confirmation bias. Initially I was just digging and investigating, so I didn't have a formed belief about glyphosate that I was trying to prove. But, in doing more research for this book I had formed that belief/theory. So, I would search and read "on both sides" of the issue. What I found was articles and sources saying GMO/glyphosate was safe, harmless, etc. But, I found issues with them as I read them. Also, with the information from the other side I was able to see certain flaws, omissions, and outright false claims or lies. Unfortunately for the public, most people lack the detailed knowledge to be able to sniff this stuff out. So, when they read these "it's harmless and fine" sources they believe them because they seem to make sense and are intentionally written to be compelling and sound very scientific, authoritative, and absolute–as well as referencing "scientific studies".

A few of these likely flaws/lies that I found have already been mentioned. Here are some of those and some other ones not yet mentioned: it doesn't hurt us because we don't have the skemitic pathway that plants do; it doesn't harm us because it doesn't get absorbed into the body and passes right through; it is only harmful in high concentrations, it is very diluted, and you are only getting tiny amounts that don't do anything bad; we tested it on rats and they were fine; we don't really put that much of it on most of the wheat crops; GMO is fundamentally the same as other food so it is fine–it is the same as hybridization that man has always done; there aren't any reputable studies showing it is bad or causes cancer. Most all of it goes into the leaves and so it doesn't pollute ground water; It doesn't stick around in the soil very long; It doesn't harm trees or wildlife. None of those are true according to multiple sources, studies, experts, my research, and my personal view and critical thinking.

Although it is a bit late, we at least are getting good science and data about GMO food, glyphosate and the potentially/likely horrible effects on human health. In fact, enough data has been accumulated, and so many people are becoming aware about this huge issue, that multiple states have tried to require GMO labeling of foods. California tried it in the past is apparently going to try it again. My state of Colorado tried it as well. The amount of funding "they" dumped into my state to fight it and run commercials about how it was safe and fine is astounding–I think it was about $14 million in advertising, and they basically bought off the public via brainwashing. However, it did a whole lot to increase awareness of the issue and many people that didn't even know what GMO/GE food was before the ballot issue now do. Even though we don't yet have GMO food labeling laws in the U.S. yet, it should be noted that many other countries do have them so that consumers can at least know it is GMO and choose accordingly.

And it isn't just average people becoming aware of the problem. Even the World Health Organization has stepped into the discussion and has stated that "glyphosate is a likely carcinogen", which means likely to cause cancer. Of course they too can't come flat out and state what they actually do know and have to say "likely" so that Monsanto doesn't take them to court or demand they recant the statement.

Monsanto has done similar things in the past and demanded a retraction of the study where the rats were fed for their entire lives– likely threatening a lawsuit if they did not. The publishing journal thoroughly investigated the study to try to find any errors or bad practices to see if a retraction was in order; They found none. They eventually did print a retraction of sorts, but it included the fact that they could find no issues with the study methodology or findings. They just said something like, "the findings weren't 100% conclusive." It should be noted that statement would be true of basically every study. In other words, the journal didn't want to do a retraction at all and sort of told readers subtly, "Yep, this study is valid and the findings legit", but no doubt they wanted to avoid a major legal battle with the giant Monsanto.

You can find many examples of this behavior by Monsanto and expect much more of it. Any/all studies, findings, articles, etc. that show GMO/glyphosate is harmful will be challenged, argued, and the people involved will be attacked. Articles will nearly instantly appear that rebut and try to debunk them. If indeed Monsanto's food and chemicals are toxic and harmful, you can bet they will go to every length and expense to block or delay the public finding out that truth.

Another huge point about the increase in actual science showing the harms, and the increasing awareness about GMOs, relates to the countries that are not allowing it. Now when a country moves to legally ban GMO's you have to understand they have to base that on some data they deem is reliable and sufficient; They review all the studies they can find and study it themselves involving multiple scientists in the many areas of health, environment, etc. In other words, they have a much higher burden of proof and need more evidence to legally ban it than you or I need to make our own personal choice.

I mentioned already that Russia wants no part of our Frankenfood. Not only have they banned any cultivation of GMO and use of glyphosate, they have completely banned any importing of GMO foods. The number of countries banning GMOs in some way has been growing at an increasing rate–it is now a trend. About 38 countries in the world now ban GMOs (either cultivation and/or importation). Recently (a vote in 2015) the majority of European Union countries decided to block cultivation of new GMOs (a vote to opt-out). Other countries are halting any more being grown, but haven't moved to ban them pending more study.

Just to give you an idea, here's a list of countries banning GMOs in some way: Germany, France, Norway, Belize, Ecuador, Peru, Venezuela, Bhutan, Kyrgyzstan, Saudi Arabia, Turkey, Algeria, Madagascar, Azerbaijan, Austria, Bosnia and Herzegovina, Bulgaria, Croatia, Cyprus, Denmark, Greece, Hungary, Italy, Latvia, Lithuania, Luxembourg, Malta, Moldova, the Netherlands, Northern Ireland, Poland, Russia, Scotland, Serbia, Slovenia, Switzerland, Ukraine, and Wales.

This long list of countries may indicate that the "cat is out of the bag" and people are finding out the truth–well, at least some of them. Many people in the U.S. (and other countries that haven't banned GMOs yet) have asked a somewhat obvious question: What do all of these countries know that we do not? However, perhaps it isn't a matter of our country not knowing it is bad stuff, but allowing it anyway. So, the question might be, "Why is it that all of those countries can protect their populations from toxins/poisons but our country won't protect its citizens, and instead chooses a mega-corporation's profits over our health?"

Now if you go back 10 years in time there were people sounding alarms and saying GMOs/glyphosate was toxic stuff and going to do a lot of damage to people's health. Some were even Monsanto and FDA scientists! But, these people were marginalized and insulted. They were made out to be paranoid health nuts, conspiracy theorists, doing "bad science and research", or just plain unintelligent and uninformed enough to tow the line that nothing was wrong with this stuff. But this has radically changed and it is becoming more widely known/believed; Additionally, more reputable "authorities", experts, scientists, and entire countries are now all saying what these supposed paranoid nuts were saying a decade ago.

We have covered a ton of ground in this chapter. Let's summarize and review briefly. My investigation into the idea that something about the wheat had changed led me onto the trail of glyphosate. By then studying glyphosate specifically, I became convinced that indeed glyphosate is the culprit in trashing the gut in ways that make us unable to digest gliadin. So, I realized/theorized it really isn't about the gluten/gliadin itself; It is about the glyphosate.

I think it was in Barrack Obama's first election run that a campaign advisor realized the most obvious issue that people wanted to be addressed; He put it this humorous way, "It's the economy stupid!"

Eventually my research led me to the revelation or theory: It's the glyphosate stupid!

Let's continue summarizing and make some conclusions. In digging into the Biochemistry and details/truth revealed about glyphosate it turns out there is substantial evidence that it has over a dozen negative impacts to our bodies. Some of these include how it trashes the various parts of the small intestine itself, as well as messing with out enzymes, sulfur pathways, and ability to use amino acids and make neurotransmitters. It also messed up our hormones that control so many functions. It is also a known chelate and depletes us of critical magnesium–the consequences of which are far reaching.

Taken together, my personal theory is that the multiple damaging effects of glyphosate cause all sorts of trouble and have the effect of creating dysfunctions in systems that all inter-relate, which has a domino effect. This leads to it being either causal or a big contributing factor to a wide number of illnesses, conditions, and chronic diseases. As it turns out, gluten sensitivity is only one of the things caused by glyphosate and GMO foods, and perhaps the least problematic of them. However, gluten sensitivity is a sure sign that our gut is in poor health and isn't working right, that we are being impacted by glyphosate, and that if we don't fix our guts then the decrease in nutrient absorption alone is going to have other negative consequences on our health. So my theory shifts things around from going "gluten free" to going "glyphosate free" and repairing the damage done.

Early on in the book I took a lot of time to discuss symptoms and how they were messengers informing us of a problem. I made the point that if we only get rid of symptoms, then the underlying problem remains, which then often gets worse over time and/or leads to other problems.

According to my theory: Now we have gotten to the bottom of things and found the core culprit behind gluten sensitivity: glyphosate. Therefore, if we only avoid gluten to remove the symptoms it causes, but do not address the core problem and issue of glyphosate, we can likely expect other and worse health problems to eventually manifest; It may also be that many people already some of these other related conditions where glyphosate is also the culprit in causing them. Therefore, it is perhaps wise to consider gluten insensitivity to be your "canary in the coal mine" that is sounding an alarm of a big danger that you need to address. But, if you stop eating glyphosate, and do some other things to heal your gut, then you will not only be able to eat gluten again, but also heal up and/or avoid many other health problems and perhaps even diseases–some of which you may already have or be in the process of developing.

There is one more key and important piece of the puzzle that will help you understand why the glyphosate and GE foods may be creating big problems for our health. However, that missing piece requires some more knowledge and information that we haven't covered yet. It will be covered right after the next short chapter and I will come back to add in this key piece that is important to really understanding what might be going on with this stuff.

You may also recall that in discussing symptoms I brought up that 400 people had self-diagnosed as being gluten sensitive, but only 14.5% of them actually were. We have discussed how glyphosate probably relates to or causes the many related conditions like IBS, leaky gut, Crohn's disease, bowel infections, magnesium deficiency, and generally trashes the gut and digestive system. These all have very similar symptoms. So, we can now see why they incorrectly self-diagnosed. However, if they had the apparent knowledge we have discussed suggesting that it's all about the glyphosate, then the cause and cure are actually the same for all of these.

Perhaps you know people that suffer from these other gut conditions, or the many other conditions and diseases that all of those charts match up nearly exactly with glyphosate/GMO. If so, you might want to consider strongly encouraging them to buy this book because the main program I will outline will probably help in fixing those things as well since they appear to have the same root cause–even if they aren't "fixed" entirely, it is very likely they will be improved and the personal overall health will improve. Who among us doesn't have family or friends suffering from that very long list of ailments? Who among us wouldn't share something that might help them? Even if you can't convince them to buy this book, you might consider buying a copy for them and giving it to them as a gift.

I have no way to directly "100% prove" my theory or what glyphosate is very probably doing to our bodies. Neither do any scientists or researchers. However, you the reader can certainly get enough information to reach your own sufficient level of conviction that will form the basis of belief that my program will indeed work to fix gluten intolerance and perhaps many other ailments as well. If you and others have success with my program, then you can post reviews on the websites of my book resellers to describe your positive results.

If enough people will do this, then perhaps it will build a long list of informal "case studies" and testimonials. This in turn will benefit many other people because they will find a solution to their suffering and ailments.

So, after you successfully complete my program, please strongly consider posting a review of any positive results. Thank you in advance.

With those two shameless self-promotions and plugs in place, let's now move on towards a solution to the problem and a pragmatic, step-by-step program to implement it.

Chapter 8: Towards a Solution

At this point let's briefly summarize everything we have covered so far in this book. Many of us used to be able to eat bread and gluten with no problem. Suddenly it happened to many of us that we now have a problem/sensitivity or intolerance for it. We found out it isn't really "gluten" that is the specific thing causing it, but instead is a particular alpha-gliadin oligopeptide. We delved into digestion and found out this gliadin is just plain hard to digest under the best of circumstances, but with the help of our marvelous gut flora/probiotics it can be done. We then reviewed and followed my investigative journey that revealed glyphosate as the likely culprit in trashing our gut health in multiple ways–including trashing our colony of gut flora.

Along the way, research about the details of glyphosate also revealed a whole host of ways it probably compromises various systems and negatively impacts our health. This glyphosate "likely culprit" was then revealed to probably be the cause or major contributor to many and varied health conditions and chronic diseases. In the end, I–and hopefully you too–realized a logical and fairly obvious operating theory, "It's the glyphosate stupid!"

We started out covering why simply going, "Gluten Free!" isn't a wise choice or approach as it only masks the symptoms and doesn't address the core problem at hand. After getting tons of details and understanding, it becomes even more clear this isn't a good approach because we also see the core problem is very likely to lead to other and worse health problems if we don't address it.

So, I've walked you through my own path of research and discovery. Let's move on to what I did next. With this new knowledge of what is at the core of the problem, or perhaps a good working theory, I then came up with a somewhat obvious general strategy that would provide a solution.

Most of this strategy and solution I have dropped in pieces along the way as we covered the various topics. Let's begin with the most obvious one: to fix gluten intolerance–and likely many other health issues–we must stop consuming the glyphosate found in the GMO foods. However, we still have major and multiple problems with our gut that need to be fixed as well.

So my solution took a general form first, and then I filled in the details. Or, you could say I came up with a strategy and then filled it in with detailed actions and solutions to cover each part of it. I also had to do some thinking about the best/proper order to do these in. Additionally, as I went into it I had to do two other things: a bit more research on the ways to implement the actions; shopping to get the required supplies, supplements, etc.

Generally speaking my strategy was this: fix the gut and stop eating GMO/glyphosate.

At first this seemed to me, and perhaps to you as well, to be fairly simple. But I found out it got a bit more complicated as I went into the next level of pragmatic and detailed actions. For example, I thought, "Okay, I need to fix or heal my gut. Hmm, how exactly do I do that?" I'd heard of doing "gut cleanses" before and how amazingly good they are and I'd even done a few methods of them. So, I figured it would be a good idea to cleanse and clear my gut out. You know, get rid of all the gunk and crud and maybe that will help a lot–flush it out. Luckily for me I had already found a pretty good gut cleansed and purchase everything to do it, which is very inexpensive and one I will share with you later.

Then I needed to figure out how to "heal" and repair my gut. This involved considering all the parts of it and what they might need because I know the body can heal itself if you give it what it needs, and also stop doing what is harming or hurting it. Mostly preventing more harm was covered by not eating more glyphosate, but there are also those 4 major foods that harm your villi. So I realized those should be avoided so the villi have a chance to repair themselves.

The next part of the gut I thought about was the gut flora because I know it is critically important for gliadin digestion. The idea of taking probiotics via supplementation occurred fairly immediately.

But, what about the intestine walls themselves and other damaged areas? Of course I also knew from my research that amino acids and magnesium would be important resources for it to begin repairing itself structurally and at the cellular level. So, I certainly needed to ensure I was getting enough of these.

I'd heard about benefits of fasting before, and one of those is that it gives your entire GI tract a "time out" and "time to heal and recover by resting" since you aren't making it work. So, that seemed like a great idea to promote my gut healing as well.

I also considered that since gluten/gliadin was currently causing inflammation and problems for my unhealthy gut, that it would be a good idea to avoid it entirely until after my gut had time to heal and I'd done everything to support that healing process. My idea and ultimate goal was that after my gut was back to a healthy state I would be able to eat gluten again, it would handle it just fine, and I would continue to not consume glyphosate to not mess it up again. Later I added in the idea that a general "gut maintenance" routine would also be a good idea to keep it healthy.

That mostly covers my general strategy, the sub-parts of it, and the actions required. After I figured this out and came up with what I thought was the best order, I then followed it step-by-step. As I said at the beginning of the book: It worked! I found that after doing this program that I could eat gluten/gliadin and had no problem with it.

Now you have a good overview of this strategy and what you too will need to do. Now we can move on to the details of each part, the best order, and cover a few other things.

Chapter 9: Glyphosate Everywhere & Not a Drop to Eat!

We are about to move into each step of my program in detail and mostly in a sequential order. Before we do that in earnest, recall from this from the last chapter: "Generally speaking my strategy was this: fix the gut and stop eating GMO/glyphosate."

I think it is best to cover the "stop eating GMO/glyphosate" part first because it is a fundamental part of the entire program. It could also be considered to be "Step 1", but also is applied to and followed during every single step of the program. Additionally, it extends and still applies after for the rest of your life even after you complete my program.

I mentioned before a general and logical approach to problem solving: stop doing what is bad/harmful and start doing what is good/helpful. Our operating theory is that glyphosate is harmful, toxic, poisonous, etc. With all we discussed about that in excruciating detail in the last chapter, I would hope you are sufficiently convinced that you don't want to be consuming this stuff anymore. But, if you aren't yet convinced that, then perhaps you should pause reading right now and do more independent research until you are.

This part of the strategy and plan of "stop eating GMOs/glyphosate" seems at first glance to be simple. It certainly isn't that many words and one might assume it would be easy and straightforward to accomplish. I wish I could tell you that is true, but unfortunately there are some complexities involved. Due to this, I'm going to provide what I think is enough information that will enable you to accomplish it.

It would be pretty easy to not eat the stuff if they put labels on all the food where it was present–wouldn't that be nice? As had been mentioned, several states have tried to require labeling, but so far we do not have it in the U.S. Some countries do have it, so if you live in one of those you have it much easier.

Since they don't label the foods elsewhere (yet), we need to have the knowledge of where all glyphosate is known or likely to be. This knowledge begins by starting with the GE (Genetically Engineered) crops themselves. After we know those crops, we can then considering where and how they get into various foods we might be eating–this part is where it gets more complicated.

For some reason, many people have this idea that all crops are GE now, or even that most of them are. In fact, there are relatively few GE crops currently being grown. The reasons for this are sensible enough:

it is incredibly expensive for GE crops to be created in the first place; they are only going to make them for certain crops that have big issues with weeds or certain pests; some crops lend themselves to the engineering while others do not or they may currently lack the technology. In other words, if farmers don't currently have a major issue growing a crop, then there is no problem to be solved, no need, and no demand for a GE version of it to be created.

So, let's look at the surprisingly short list of the primary GE crops currently being grown–note that there are many more than these that have been approved, but aren't being grown for a variety of reasons. There are also some GE crops that are being grown, but not very much of them. Therefore, we will take a look at the biggest three first (by acreage planted), then the top 9 by adding 6 more, and then mention two other new ones.

Top 3 GE crops: Field Corn, Soy, and Cotton

6 more making the top 9 GE crops: Sweet Corn, Sugar Beets, Canola (Rapeseed), Rainbow Papaya, Alfalfa, and Summer Squash

New GE crops: Apple that doesn't brown (Fall 2017), a new "bruise free" potato (2016).

At first glance that certainly isn't very long of a list. You might read it over and think for a moment that going glyphosate free is going to be pretty simple. For example, "Well, I don't eat cotton or alfalfa, I can stop eating corn, I'm not into tofu (made of soy), I never cared for beets anyway, and I can eat other squashes." If only it were that simple!

We will have to next investigate where and how this short list of crops gets used and eaten. As we do, I'll add in some important statistics as well. I'm not just going to give lists of how the crops get used and ways you consume them for educational purposes or to make some point–although there is a major point. Instead, this is giving you specific and valuable information that you need to learn in order to go glyphosate free. In other words, I'm giving you the list of all the foods you cannot be eating–at least not if made with GMOs/GE crops.

Let's start with the field corn. In the U.S. in 1996 about 3% of the acres were growing GE field corn. As of 2014, that grew to about 85%. But, maybe this "field corn" is just the stuff they feed cows and we just eat the "sweet corn"–unfortunately not. They use this field corn to make high-fructose corn syrup, which has almost entirely replaced sugar in soda pop, candy, and most processed foods–they also make other sweeteners out of it. This means dang near anything sweet probably has GE corn at its base. You probably didn't think about eating corn when you drink a soda.

In addition, they make tons of corn oil out of it, which is a major oil people and restaurants alike use–or it is blended into many "vegetable oils". Of course many baked goods and processed foods contain oil. But, this also means that dang near any fried foods are sources of glyphosate. Consider how many fried foods people eat and how much we love them. French fries, onion rings, fried shrimp, fried chicken and wings, and things they coat with breading and fry like fish, tempura vegetables, etc.

They also use field corn in cereals, which means you (and/or children) are getting it for breakfast. Of course some cereals are made from wheat (or a mixture with corn), but we already know about glyphosate getting into wheat. Then you have things like corn starch being made from it as well as corn meal (think about the stuff on the bottom of the pizza crust), which again make their way into many/most all baked goods and tons of processed foods. Of course there are also the many things we know are made from corn directly like corn chips, corn tortillas, tamales, Cheetos, etc.

From all of these, you can begin to see how just the GE crop of field corn gets used in literally thousands of individual foods or products we eat. The two primary ways it makes its way into other foods are certainly the corn oil and the high-fructose corn syrup. But even those two mean that thousands of foods become "potentially contaminated and toxic". Those are a lot of foods you have to cut out to go glyphosate free. However, we will discuss alternatives so that you can still eat baked foods and even fried foods.

We are nearly finished with field corn. But field corn is indeed fed to cows, poultry, and other livestock. We previously covered how glyphosate finds its way into animal tissues and bones. Many of these we consume direct or indirectly. Consider what they are making that chicken stock from; Hint, it isn't from boiling the expensive breasts. The field corn glyphosate might end up in eggs and meat products. Of course we don't think about eating corn when we have chicken soup, a cookie, Jello, or a piece of cake, but we actually are. You need to get this general concept of the source GE crop being used to make other products/foods that we ordinarily wouldn't think about as being at all related.

Summarizing about field corn, we see a prime example of how glyphosate works its way down from the crop to a huge variety of end products we consume. See how it isn't just as simple as, "Well, I'll stop eating corn on the cob and canned corn"?

Before we move on to soy, let me add two other small things about field corn. You might recall I mentioned "other sweeteners" they make from corn. The big one is maltodextrin. If you read labels you are familiar with it, but may not know what it really is. In short, it is the starch (simple sugar/glucose) that is extracted from several vegetables. As such, they are fundamentally sugar, although they are chemically slightly different–sugar has glucose in it. Due to this, they are legally not considered "sugar" and so they are commonly and widely used in things that say, "sugar free" or "low in sugar". This is very deceptive because they are just long chains of glucose (what you have and use as blood sugar); As such, they jack up your blood sugar level even faster and more than sugar does. Yes, they will make you gain weight, or develop insulin resistance and/or type II diabetes like sugar does. They make maltodextrin from corn, rice, potato starch, or wheat. So, if a label says it has maltodextrin in it, you may very well be getting a dose of glyphosate if it is made from corn or wheat. I do not know if during the refining process the glyphosate is stripped out and removed. However, table sugar is similarly refined and is known to have traces of glyphosate in it from the sugar beets, so it seems likely. In the end, because it is fundamentally unhealthy anyway, I'd strongly recommend avoiding it. Note that many "Stevia" products that are sold as a healthy alternative to sugar are actually mostly made of maltodextrin, which makes them no better. Stevia itself is fine, not sugar in any way, and healthy; You just need to get the pure goopy form that is a bit less convenient and be sure to read the label very carefully to ensure it is pure stevia only.

Speaking of "distilled", whiskey and vodka are normally made from corn. However, the distillation process does not leave any glyphosate behind because it is "too heavy" to go up in the vapor during distillation. Many of these alcohols are also double or triple distilled. When you go on my program you don't want to be drinking alcohol–or very little of it–because it can feed the candida in your gut and crowd out the good gut flora. However, after you heal your gut you can drink these in moderation without concerning yourself with them containing glyphosate. While we are on the subject, gliadin is also in barley; Of course barley is used in beer. So, during the time you are going gluten free until you complete the program, beer is either off limits or you can actually now buy "gluten free beer".

Let's now take a look at soy. As of 2014, 94% of all soy grown in the U.S. is GE soy. You might think you don't eat soy, but you very likely consume quite a bit without knowing it. Soybeans are used to make soybean oil, which is typically just labeled and marketed as simply "vegetable oil". As previously noted, some vegetable oils sold are mixtures–commonly corn and soy, but sometimes with canola also. Again this means baked goods, fried foods, and many processed foods will have glyphosate from soy in them.

But, there is another thing they make from soybeans called, "soy lecithin". If you ever read the label of ingredients for packaged and processed foods then you no doubt have seen it listed in basically all of them–start reading labels generally, and notice this soy lecithin stuff. What is this stuff and why do they use and put it in everything they make? The short answer is this stuff is very useful in making commercial foods in a variety of ways. It is an emulsifier, which means it will allow oil and water to mix together when ordinarily they won't.

So, soy lecithin gets used in all tons of creamy salad dressings, mayonnaise, reduced fat butter spreads and margarine, or other foods that have lots of oil in them. They also use it as an emulsifier in chocolate, which makes it all smooth. They even put soy lecithin in things like granola bars and flavored tea bags–and thousands of other products–because it stabilizes the fat emulsions so it doesn't go bad and has longer shelf life. There are other reasons they use it to make things such as it reducing the stickiness so their products are easier to work with. Soy lecithin is also a surfactant, which means it reduces the surface tension and makes it easier and faster to add water–think fast processing and no lumps. So, they put it in nearly everything they make that is in batter form, or add it to things like cake mixes that you are going to make into a batter.

You can see it has tons of very valuable uses to the food manufacturers, but most health experts agree it is nasty and unhealthy stuff. Soy in general is well known to mess with your hormones. But when we add in the GE component, this soy lecithin becomes another source of glyphosate exposure and rather hidden consumption. Start looking for it on labels and you will realize that between it and the vegetable oil that you are indeed getting lots of soy–and glyphosate from it. While there may not be tons of soy lecithin in any one product or serving, the fact that it is in damn near any packaged or processed food means that the amount adds up and accumulates. Additionally, we know that even small amounts of glyphosate are likely to do big ugly things in our bodies.

I will also mention a very sad and tragic use of soy: they put it in baby formula! Every baby formula supplied by the government's WIC program (Women, Infants, and Children) has GE products in it. It is a long and tangled story outside our scope, but studies on rats have also shown that newborns of parents have decreased fertility in addition to other issues. But it gets worse. When they then have litters, the litter size is decreased and there are more deformities and problems. After they got to the 4th generation of feeding rats the Frankenfood, no rats were able to reproduce–100% sterile. By the way, infertility rates in the U.S. also match up on graphs nearly exactly with the increased rate of glyphosate and GE crops–isn't that fascinating? So, if you happen to have a baby and can't breast feed, be damn sure you know what is in the infant formula you use. And please don't feed your kids candy, soda, and GE breakfast cereals! They are innocent, don't have the choice of what they eat, and you are the one that has to have the knowledge and make the healthy choices for them! Don't feed them Frankenfood!

Lastly on soy, they also feed it to livestock and poultry. This of course means some of the glyphosate is going to end up in their tissues, some of which we consume. Or, it may end up in things like the eggs in some amount. It is a rather bizarre but true connection to realize that when you are eating a chicken sandwich you are actually indirectly eating some soy. The same can be said of eating a French fry, cookie, cake, or doughnut. Again we see an example of how glyphosate works its way down from the crop to an end product we consume.

Let's now move on to the last of the big 3: cotton. We find GE cotton acreage to again be about 90%, which is similar to corn and soy. At first glance I actually thought to myself, "Well I sure as heck don't eat cotton!" But, as with soy, you are basically eating GE cotton without knowing it. "I'm eating cotton? You must be crazy!" you must be thinking. Allow me to explain.

Cotton makes seeds like nearly every plant. Now of course they use cotton to make clothing, but they have no use or desire to have the seeds in there. So, they use the seeds to make cottonseed oil. Cottonseed oil has a colorful history, but suffice it to say they had lots of seeds lying around, they were illegally dumping them in rivers, and a general oil shortage occurred. So, they thought to themselves, "Surely there can be some use for all of these cotton seeds that we can think of and then sell the stuff to make a buck?" Enter cottonseed oil.

Cottonseed oil, like many oils, doesn't start out to be particularly unhealthy. Unfortunately, an inexpensive way to process it is to hydrogenate it. It starts out as 70% unsaturated fatty acids, but after it is fully hydrogenated, it end up being 94% saturated fat. As you may or may not be aware, it is common thought that unsaturated fat is actually healthy, but saturated fat is the "bad fat" that trashes your heart and arteries. Sources such as the Mayo Clinic and American Heart Association are really down on it, advise against getting much of it, and doctors have been telling people to avoid it for decades.

This same process of making hydrogenated oils is also done for the corn oil, soy/vegetable oil, and many other oils. Some oils are also processed with nasty hexane gunk. Plastic is made from petroleum/oil. What they do to these oils basically turns them into plastic in terms of how your body cannot deal with them. Things like butter substitutes spreads, margarine, mayonnaise, salad dressings, etc. are chocked full of this Frankenplastic. You wouldn't chew up and eat plastic would you? Well, then you have to stop eating this unhealthy saturated fat Frakenplastic crud!

They do not have to hydrogenate the oils–they just do it to save money/costs. The oils can be extracted by mashing and squishing them mechanically–"expeller-pressed". You want to switch to using pure sunflower oil (there are no GE sunflowers) and one that is also expeller-pressed. Sunflower oil actually has about a dozen health benefits, a good taste, and is well suited to many uses including withstanding frying temperatures. Coconut oil, safflower oil, and olive oil are also good non-GE alternatives.

However, recently it has been found that many popular olive oil companies have been cheating and mixing in other oils that are GE oils; So, be sure to research that if you are going to get/use olive oil. Another alternative, if you can find it, is a non-GMO canola oil that is expeller-pressed. Personally I use coconut oil mainly as a supplement of healthy fats, some pure olive oil for certain needs, and then expeller-pressed sunflower oil for everything else.

Okay, so generally speaking this hydrogenated cottonseed oil is bad for your health to begin with. Now add in the facts that it is one of those GE crops where they put in the Bt toxin and also made it herbicide resistant as well–"Roundup Ready" is what they call them. So, you are getting the glyphosate and also those Bt bacteria that rots the guts out of the pests and kills them–and possibly rots our guts out as well according to certain studies.

Back to the colorful history, Proctor and Gamble cornered the market on cottonseed oil and invented a new product they marketed as a supposedly healthier "lard substitute". I'm sure you have heard of this product: Crisco. But this probably isn't the Crisco you grew up on because that was from 1911 to about 1944. A bit prior to Crisco, a food chemist named David Wesson came out with a cottonseed oil product: Wesson Oil. Between the two, cottonseed oil was the most widely used oil in the U.S. for over 30 years. In fact, we used so much that the supply suffered and prices rose. At that point, soybean oil became cheaper and took over for a while. They then switched Crisco over to being made of soybean oil.

So, where does this oil make its way into our foods? They like to use cottonseed oil in salad dressing and mayonnaise due to its initial flavor and also because the oil won't change flavor after aging–back to their greed and need for long shelf life. Currently cottonseed oil is significantly less expensive than canola or other oils that can withstand well the high heat of frying and do so repeatedly. Therefore, it has been widely used in making potato chips, other fried snack foods, and is a very popular frying oil for restaurants.

So, although you don't eat cotton, you are indirectly eating it if you have snack foods, potato chips, eat certain mayonnaise brands, or eat fried foods out at restaurants. We now see another large group of foods that inherit and contain glyphosate.

There are two more short points about cottonseed oil. Once again it turns out it is used in animal feed, and we know what that means. There is also an interesting fact that untreated cottonseed oil is used as a pesticide. They have been putting it on the bark of apple trees because it kills a particular moth that burrows into the trees and can kill them. Oils, including vegetable oils, have actually been used for centuries as a pesticide–this might give us some pause for concern. As it turns out, cottonseed is the most powerful pesticide of any vegetable oil.

Now that we have covered the top 3 GE crops, it should be crystal clear to you that they end up directly and indirectly into thousands of foods, products, and meals we eat. Market Watchers estimate that upwards of 70% of processed foods in the supermarket contain GE ingredients. So even just these 3 GE crops turn out to put glyphosate into multiple food groups/types and thousands of products. That was my point in making the title of this chapter: "Chapter 9: Glyphosate Glyphosate everywhere, and not a drop to Eat!" The stuff is literally everywhere, and you shouldn't eat a drop of it! But don't despair; we will discuss how to get plenty of food without the glyphosate.

Two chapters ago I mentioned a key and important piece of the puzzle. I said we needed some more information to understand how it fits in. We have now covered most all of that information: glyphosate and GE ingredients find their way into dang near everything. So, let's insert this key piece and come to an important understanding about what it means to us. What is happening to people is that they are getting a little bit of glyphosate from a huge number of sources, foods, meals, drinks, etc.

The revelation or understanding is that while we aren't getting huge doses of glyphosate from any one source or meal, we are getting many small doses over a long period of time–over many months and

years. It is like taking just a little bit of poison every day–one small dose won't kill you, but eventually it is going to catch up to you and manifest something substantial. So, the consequence of frequent and nearly continuous intake of glyphosate is that it very probably takes a cumulative toll on our health and multiple systems in our bodies; We discussed how it apparently and literally accumulates in various parts of our body, and this happens over time and small exposures being adding together; We eat a little bit of it at a time–and that likely only does a little damage–but as we keep eating it over the months and years, any potential damage and harm gets larger and more significant.

This understanding also empowers us to be able to see through the many claims and common rebuttals of those people and groups that attempt to say glyphosate and GE foods are harmless and fine for us to eat. Nearly every article along these lines I have read will point out something about the "PPM" or "PPB" (parts-per-million or per billion), which is the way they measure how much glyphosate is in things. Basically they claim that since there are such tiny amounts of it that it isn't enough to be harmful. Again, the flawed logic of this is easily seen when you realize they are basically saying, "It's just a little bit of poison, so don't worry about it." The fact that they actually have established legal limits for how much glyphosate can be in stuff should give you pause for concern–they are flat out saying they know it is poisonous and toxic, but that they think a certain amount of it is acceptable.

Again, the one counter-point to their ridiculous use of the PPM/PPB thing is that while it may be just a little in one particular ingredient, product, food, meal, etc, we are eating so many of these on a regular basis over time that it doesn't end up being a "little bit of poison" anymore; It adds up to "a lot of poison continuously ingested and accumulating over time". A second counter-point is that there are multiple studies showing things like even very tiny amounts well under the allowed PPB actually do damage our organs and cause harm; Or recall the rat study with the Bt toxin where 800 times the dosage of pure Bt didn't cause harm, but the 1/800th dosage inside the potatoes did do lots of harm. Therefore, "it's just a tiny bit and won't harm you" appears to be disproven and is patently false on two accounts: a tiny bit is harmful; we aren't just getting a tiny bit, but a large amount when we consider that glyphosate is in dang near everything these days and we consume it regularly and over a period of years or decades.

As a reminder, the main offenders are all of the oils made from the big 3, anything that these oils get used in, the soy lecithin found everywhere, and the high-fructose corn syrup that is now the primary "sugar" and sweetener. We can add table sugar to this list of main offenders because it is made from GE sugar beets.

When you consider some processed/packaged, ready made, or restaurant foods, it is easy to see they may actually contain all of these. A package of candy or a packaged frozen dinner may have corn, wheat, high-fructose corn syrup, soy lecithin, and oil. A fast food meal may have wheat in a bun, glyphosate residue in the meat, sugar in the ketchup, high-fructose corn syrup in the soda, and GE oil used to cook the French fries. Viewing these "foods" in light of what we have discussed and theorized, they appear to be something like a Frankenfood soup, or an evil witch's brew and poisonous concoction made of multiple vile and harmful GE ingredients. There are many examples of this witch's brew and multiple GE ingredients included "all in one meal/package".

Imagine if a report came out and said, "Glyphosate found in hamburger buns!" You can see how a GE advocate would be recruited to rebut this and write an article saying something nonsensical like, "Well there is only a tiny amount of residue in a wheat bun–just a few PPB; There's no cause for concern here." Meanwhile, they are totally neglecting and failing to consider the entire meal that we just discussed that has much more glyphosate than just what is in the bun. They would also not be considering the cereal the person had for breakfast, or what their dinner meal was, or how many other sodas they drank in the day, or how much sugar they put in their coffee, etc. Instead of believing their bunk about some small PPB in one thing, consider something more like "total glyphosate intake for the entire day", and then add that up to the total in a month, year, and over the course of 10 years!

Let's get back to the packaged and processed food. Based upon how we see GE ingredients in nearly all of it, some general advice to avoid buying foods with glyphosate is to not buy packaged foods, ready made foods, processed foods, etc. In other words, instead you want to buy whole foods in their original form, or only those that you can read the ingredients and know they do not contain the things we have just discussed. Grocery stores usually follow a similar layout: the inner isles are processed foods and around the three sides you have produce, meat, and then dairy. So, a general thing to try to do is to walk around and shop only the outside walls/isles of the store; Of course there are some non-food products in the isles you will need.

Another general piece of advice is to avoid most all restaurants and in particular fast food places. Interestingly, the major chain restaurant Chipotle has decided to remove all GE foods from its restaurant and all the food they serve! So, I guess you can go out to eat there; Other restaurants may follow suit. Also, if you look around and ask people, you will very likely find very healthy/organic mom-and-pop restaurants in your town. So, you can still eat out at restaurants, but you need to be informed and conscientious about doing so.

Another crop we can discuss is the rapeseed, or more commonly it is called Canola. It became very popular as canola oil due to supposedly being healthier than other oils. The problem with that hype/marketing is threefold: that nonsense came from the people making and selling it; it is usually hydrogenated too, which undoes any original benefits; it is a GE crop so it has the glyphosate in it. If you had nature's version of canola and expeller-pressed it, then it might be healthier, but that's not what they are primarily selling and pushing onto an unsuspecting and uneducated public.

We don't need to say much more about canola that we don't already know. People buy and use it for baking and frying. It makes its way into multiple products; For example they now market mayonnaise "With Canola Oil!" to lure you into buying that type because of the hype/lies about it being healthier. It too is fed to livestock. The point here is only to make you aware of it being a GE crop and to not buy, use, or expose yourself to it.

Our last rather big GE crop we need to discuss is sugar beets. No, they aren't just the beets you eat, which I wouldn't eat if you paid me anyway. They call them "sugar" beets because they are what they use to make white table sugar from. So, anything that has sugar in it is now going to pass along the glyphosate. And yes, even though it is highly refined, they have found glyphosate residue in sugar. Consider how many foods have sugar in them. Now consider how much sugar people add to drinks, other things, or use in baking. Ponder that a moment and let it sink in.

I've read articles over the years with statistics similar to these: "Two hundred years ago, the average American ate only 2 pounds of sugar a year. In 1970, we ate 123 pounds of sugar per year. Today, the average American consumes almost 152 pounds of sugar in one year." Now those statistics include all forms of sugar such as the corn syrup, fruits, honey, etc. Even so, I did some rough Math based upon pie charts and it comes out to more than 50% of it is white table sugar. That means the average American eats about 75 pounds of GE sugar beet sugar with glyphosate a year! A major portion of the rest is the GE corn-based high-fructose corn syrup. Ponder these statistics and facts about sugar and the GE table sugar for a few moments and really let it sink in.

Sugar is used in many things just to tweak the flavor even if the product doesn't really taste sweet. Ketchup is loaded with the stuff. But if it does taste sweet then you know that it either has sugar and/or high-fructose corn syrup in it–and/or possibly maltodextrin.

You might wonder if the glyphosate really makes it all the way down into the foods when the GE crop is processed into oils, sugars, lecithin, etc. The apparent answer is that it absolutely does. Multiple groups have taken the products and tested them for glyphosate. One group found, "…shocking levels of glyphosate contamination in popular American foods, including Cheerios, Doritos, Oreos, Goldfish and Ritz crackers and Stacy's Pita Chips. Levels found in these products are well above the levels found by independent peer-reviewed studies which show that ultra-low levels of glyphosate can cause organ damage starting at 0.1 parts per billion (ppb). This is 1,750 times lower than what the EPA currently claims is safe. The highest levels detected were found in General Mills' Original Cheerios, which were simply off the charts, at 1,125.3 ppb or nearly twice the level considered potentially harmful according to the latest scientific research in a single serving for young children." Most all of the breakfast cereals contain glyphosate; Again, please don't feed your children these Frankencereals and don't eat them yourself either. Note that apparently Monsanto themselves owns General Mills–hmm.

Based upon what we've already discussed several times, what do you think happened when the above testing for glyphosate residue in grocery products came out and was published? Of course there immediately followed multiple articles trying to debunk or minimize the findings of the tests. I read one of them and it basically said two things: Well, it is such tiny PPB that it is not going to hurt and is safe; They only found it because they were looking for it; If they had been looking for some other pesticide or herbicide they would have found those too.

The first part we already covered and know it is bullpucky and false on two accounts. But, how retarded is that last statement? Firstly, of course they were looking for it; That was their point and what they wanted to find out: is it making it all the way down into the end products we consume? Secondly, to say that somehow it doesn't matter just because there are other toxic chemicals in our food is utterly nonsensical and illogical. It is like saying, "Yeah, you found our poison in these products, but that is no big deal because there are other poisons in them too." In the end, it shows once again the intentional and ongoing effort to slow down or block people from getting to the truth of the GE food situation.

Let's wrap up with some of the other GE crops. Alfalfa is the only other major crop we haven't covered. Yeah, we certainly don't eat it– at least not directly. But naturally it is a primary feed for cattle and we eat those; We know glyphosate ends up in bovine/cattle tissues–and also the vaccines made from their gelatin. This also would include Jello, gummy bears, and many other gelatin containing products. But since the main use is cattle feed, this brings beef into the mix of foods with some level of glyphosate contamination/residue.

The rest of the GE crops are easy enough to avoid and don't make their way into other foods. Don't eat the sweet corn unless it's local and you know it isn't GE; If you must eat corn, then a farmer's market or local farmer can be a good option if you can verify it isn't GE sweet corn. The rainbow papaya is only grown in Hawaii; there are other papayas to eat so we can avoid them–besides they don't get glyphosate on them because they were just engineered to resist a particular pest. The GE summer squash is just one variety grown in California. We can eat other squashes or find local suppliers the same as with sweet corn.

We have one new apple to avoid if we want to that is called the "Arctic apple", and there are thousands of apples varieties to choose from. Additionally, it seems they just altered the one gene that makes them turn brown–therefore they aren't putting glyphosate on them nor inserted the Bt toxin. They likely did the same thing with the "bruise free" potato. We can also largely ignore these because they are new and historically GE potatoes never caught on due to fast food restaurants rejecting them. We can just stick to the potatoes we have been eating and it is highly unlikely you would even encounter these new ones.

<u>Summary and Review</u>: That concludes covering that relatively short list of GE crops. We know the main offenders are the oils, table sugar, high-fructose corn syrup, soy lecithin, and all of the foods these get used in. So, stop eating all of those as well as the direct foods such as the field corn in cereals, soymilk, corn chips, etc. We know snacks and candies have multiple GE ingredients, so stop eating those. We know the same is true about most all processed foods, packaged foods, mixes, prepared or ready-to-eat foods, frozen dinners/entrees, fast food, and most restaurants. Our general strategy is to simply stop buying these types of foods and instead switch to whole foods and eat them whole or prepare them into meals ourselves.

This is the first step: going glyphosate free. It is also something you need to do through all steps of my program and after the program on an ongoing basis. You need to do this because we know it is the likely culprit causing the core problem. You can't fix gluten sensitivity and improve your health without doing this, and you certainly can't heal your gut if you continue to pump poison into it.

It may be a tall order to get off of GE foods and glyphosate, but it is well worth the effort because it will radically improve your health in another way: you will fundamentally improve your diet and be eating healthier because you will be switching to natural foods, whole foods, and organic foods. You will also likely be doing a lot more cooking and preparing of your own meals, which is the best way to know what all is going into your body and to have total control over it.

In keeping with the general concept of, "Stop the bad and start the good", I think we now need to cover what you can eat. The list of stuff you can no longer eat is quite long and it may seem there isn't anything left to eat, but that is far from true. So, let's now get some general and specific ideas about how to "start the good", or how to start eating healthy and GE/glyphosate free.

Chapter 10: What the heck can I Eat?

Since we have just eliminated 70% of the things found in the grocery store from your diet, we need to cover what the heck you are now going to eat instead of that crapola and packages of noxious witch's brew. Eating out at restaurants is also greatly limited. But, you should know by now that you need to get off of the GE/Glyphosate, so you need the alternatives. There are two basic approaches or strategies to accomplishing this goal.

The first of these is to basically try to buy what you can determine isn't GE. You can do this based upon the knowledge of what is GE we just covered. For example, since there is no such thing as GE lettuce or russet potatoes, you know you can buy and eat those. As mentioned already, you can generally and mainly switch to whole foods, which are foods in the same form as the Earth or nature make them. There can be some exceptions if they are minimally processed, or if you know for a fact they don't have GE ingredients in them.

Certainly people survived for thousands of years and ate many things that weren't ready-made, processed, or genetically engineered. Therefore, it may involve some changes being made, but we know it certainly can be done. Again, in general you want to shop at the grocery store by walking around the outside walls and isles to get your foodstuffs. Hit the produce isle. Since the list of actual produce that is GE is so tiny, it is easy to avoid them and you can basically buy any fruits and vegetables.

What else naturally grows that you can eat whole? How about seeds and nuts? These are great sources of protein and healthy fats and oils as well. Raw ones are typically better as some nutrient benefits are destroyed by roasting the seeds/nuts. Sunflower seeds, cashews, and almonds are particularly good choices. In my supermarket there are tons of seeds and nuts near the end of the produce isle. So, you can fill up your cart with lots of vegetables, a few fruits, and seeds/nuts.

What else grows, is non-GMO, and something you can eat in unprocessed form? How about grains? We are going to have to stay off gluten/gliadin for a while, so wheat is out. But rice isn't GE, so you can get some rice. Oatmeal is a good grain and is high fiber, which will help with your gut cleansing. There are other grains that are healthy as well such as amaranth, and many others. So, buy some grains to cook up and some oatmeal you can have for breakfast instead of that crap in a box that they tested positive for glyphosate.

The last major food group that the Earth directly makes is the legumes or beans. They are great sources of protein/amino acids. They also have lots of minerals, vitamins, fiber, and more good stuff in them such as healthy fats and oils. In addition, there are like a gazillion varieties of beans. Now you don't necessarily want to go buy them in a can–especially if they are in some ready-to-eat meal form. But buying the straight beans alone in cans is okay. There are studies and evidence that the linings of the cans have a noxious chemical that bleeds into the contents; So, you might consider the dried beans or frozen ones instead. Dried beans are incredibly cheap, but you have to soak them forever before using them, or slow cook them in a crock-pot for a long time.

This then leaves animal products. Of course here we need to be a bit careful due to the potential glyphosate residue. But, you can usually find organic and/or organic grass-fed beef and hamburger in the supermarket these days. If not, a health food store will have them. Some people will buy a grass-fed cow and have it processed and freeze it; many will go in with someone or several people and get 1/2 or 1/4, etc.

Organic has become pretty popular, so you can find organic meats, organic eggs, and organic cheese. This then wraps up how you can make your trip mostly around the store and get GE/glyphosate free whole foods: vegetables, nuts, seeds, grains, beans, meet, poultry, eggs, cheese, etc. Notice that most all of these are going to require some preparation or cooking to be done to turn them into a meal. There's no more zapping some frozen FrankenTVdinner in the microwave or popping a chemical brew frozen pizza into the oven.

However, there are some ready-to-eat or prepared meal things that might actually be free of GE ingredients. You can browse around and become really good at reading the ingredient labels. From this point forward you need to know precisely what is going into your mouth, and you always need to read the ingredients of any product you buy. One of the primary ways you can get basically a ready-to-eat or quick to prepare meal is to buy ones that are specifically labeled as "organic", but there are some complications about the various labels we need to cover.

This is actually the second basic strategy to avoid all GE/glyphosate: buying and eating organic foods. However, you will encounter a variety of labels: "Organic Ingredients", "Organic", "Certified Organic", and "100% Organic" or "Certified 100% Organic".

Let's start with the best, most informative, and the label you really want on products that you buy: 100% Certified Organic. This means that 100% of everything in the product must follow the strict rules. It also means that the producer has gone through a long and detailed process to become certified–initially inspected, processes and land examined, and end products examined periodically to ensure continued compliance. The crops cannot be grown with synthetic fertilizers (which includes glyphosate/Roundup), synthetic pesticides or sewage sludge, and it means that organic crops cannot be genetically engineered or irradiated. Animal products that are certified organic must eat only organically grown feed (without animal byproducts) and can't be treated with synthetic hormones or antibiotics, animals must have access to the outdoors, and ruminants (hoofed animals, including cows) must have access to pasture, and animals cannot be cloned. The bottom line is that Certified Organic means no GE crops of any kind anywhere in the process and no glyphosate/Roundup was used either.

Then next best label is "Certified Organic". It means that 95-99% of the ingredients and contents must follow the same rules above. But, they allow a bit of wiggle room because certain products simply cannot be made to the 100% level due to the complexity and strictness of the rules. For example, perhaps the product is mainly all organic, but they added some milk that was irradiated. This should be considered a pretty darn good label, especially as compared to no label at all or a known GE product. For example, there could be no way that hamburger could be labeled certified organic and be made from cows eating GMO grains because it would be way beyond the percentages allowed. But, in these products you may find some small amounts of things like the soy lecithin or a tad of sugar, corn syrup, etc. Of course it would depend upon the product and this is another good reason to always read the ingredients so you can spot such things.

Next we have "Organic". As far as I can tell this means the same as certified organic in that it must be at least 95% organic. However, this is apparently something like an honor system and it hasn't been through formal certification. The certification process is long, expensive, and difficult. So, a company may be working its way through that process, but just not yet completed it. Or, a producer may be too small to afford it. I suppose technically anyone could analyze the organic product and if it isn't up to the standards they could sue the company for false advertising. But, with many companies marketing and wanting to be organic, this label becomes a bit questionable. Even so, it would seem a far cry better than buying products that you know are GE/glyphosate ones.

Just for the sake of completeness, there are also labels you will see that say "natural", "all natural", or "made from natural ingredients". These are basically meaningless and just marketing tactics. It only means there are supposedly no synthetic and artificial things in them.

But there are no specific legal requirements or enforcements for these. Consider that gasoline is made from "all natural ingredients" too!

Having covered the labeling, let's get into this second general strategy. So instead of trying to sort through every food and products to see if it has GE/glyphosate in it, we can instead take the simple approach of buying organic foods and that right there tells us it isn't Frankenfood. This greatly simplifies things. Also, as I had mentioned, this will allow you to fill in your shopping and eating with some pre-made meals and products when you can find alternative ones that are organic–or hopefully 100% Certified Organic.

Organics are becoming popular enough that you can buy many of the types of foods you already eat that aren't whole foods. For example, on the shelf you can find organic versions of ketchup, peanut butter, butter, eggs, cheese, soup, bread, chips and snacks, etc. Lays recently came out with a whole line of their snacks called "Simply". You can get Simply Lays potato chips that are organic potatoes, sea salt, and fried in expeller-pressed sunflower oil! No other ingredients at all. They have Simply versions of Tostitos, Cheetos, etc. Stronger consider a switch to those for kids.

You don't have to buy everything organic because you know that many foods don't have GE ingredients or glyphosate in them anyway. However, you can use the "buy organic" strategy when you know you are buying things that normally are GE. For example corn chips, meat, dairy, snacks, mayonnaise, dressings, etc. Or for all those things that have the oils, sugar, high-fructose corn syrup, and soy lecithin in them. Again you can read labels to help out with this. At home you might pick up some product you normally buy and read the label and find one or more GE ingredients. Throw it in the trash and make a note to buy an organic alternative of it next time.

Even though supermarkets are stocking way more organic products, you may not be able to find everything you want. Also, they tend to be lacking in selection. A solution to this is to get what you can at the supermarket, but then also make a trip to a local health food store. There you will find a wide selection and in general much less of the Frankenfood to even have to watch out for in the first place.

Some people may claim they are too busy to cook very often. Some don't even shop that much and/or rarely cook. Well, they pay the price with their health. But there are some really positive points and smart things you can do if you are one of these people. You can make many foods in a batch. For example, you might spend an hour on a day off making a nice stew with potatoes, onions, organic chicken stock or cream of chicken soup, amaranth, rice, and maybe some organic ham or bacon. You can eat off of this several days in a week, and/or freeze half of it. You can take it to work and eat it for lunch–just take it in glass and never microwave plastic! Salads don't take too long to prepare, but even so they keep pretty well; You can make a big salad for dinner and have leftovers for lunch the next day or dinner the next evening. You can make an organic, grass-fed meatloaf and have great leftovers. These are just a few examples, the point is that with a bit of planning and thinking about it, you can find time to cook great meals and avoid the instant/processed ones or restaurants.

If you have kids, what a great way to spend quality time together and also give them a great education. As a child, my favorite thing to do was to help my mom in the kitchen. You might even come to enjoy and love cooking–it might become a new hobby and passion. Cooking for yourself (and/or your family) and using whole foods can be a creative challenge; You often find yourself finding, making, and enjoying meals that are new to you. There are two more key points: the main thing is that you are getting off the glyphosate and that is likely one of the best things you can do for your overall health; in place of that, you will be eating whole foods and organic foods that are fundamentally healthier than processed foods and restaurants. Both of these lead to a feeling of satisfaction and pride, which somehow makes the meals taste better too.

Pragmatically speaking, as soon as you have read this chapter is the time to start acting on it. By this I mean to of course stop eating GE/glyphosate. But, I also mean to stop buying the stuff and bringing it into your home. While this may seem extreme or wasteful, I would also strongly encourage you to go through your cupboard and refrigerator and throw out all of the stuff you now know is trashing your body–it is trash. This is very helpful because you may be tempted to cheat, snack, or somehow eat that stuff even knowing what you now know. But, if it isn't in your house you can't do that. If you have a spouse, significant other, or roommates then maybe you don't have to throw it out. However, consider that you are just allowing them to eat the poison that you yourself won't eat.

Also, if you have children then it is my strong opinion it isn't ethical to have them eat it up as if they are being your garbage disposal. I mean it is technically a poison; Do you really feel okay about knowingly feeding your child poison? You might have to have a family meeting, or you can just make the changes without saying much about it and see how that goes. Kids will certainly complain without their favorite cereals, sodas, snacks, candy, etc. But hey, I never got any of that as a child and the glyphosate issue notwithstanding you ought to know that most of that stuff isn't healthy for them. So, perhaps this is the perfect time to clean up their diets, gem them off the sugar and junk food, and start healing their bodies as well. I suppose you could wait until after they get obese, ADHD, type II diabetes, autism, gluten sensitivity, etc. and then make a change.

Also, maybe you can involve your children in this entire process; They can read this book; Help shop and read labels and ingredients; and help prepare and cook healthy glyphosate-free meals. Most kids love to learn and to help out their parents–use that to your advantage and theirs as well.

Summary and Review: It may have seemed that after seeing how glyphosate is everywhere that there would be nothing left to eat anymore. However, by using and combining two basic strategies, along with your knowledge of GE foods and ingredients, you can find plenty to eat. Use your knowledge about GE to avoid the processed Frankenfoods and directly GE crops; Instead use the "buy whole foods" strategy to get healthy foods the Earth makes for the foods you know aren't GE; Do a lot more cooking and preparing of your own food. Then use the "buy organic" to fill in the rest for foods you know would otherwise be GE and also to be able to have some processed or prepared foods for convenience. Switch to using expeller-pressed sunflower, safflower, pure olive, and/or coconut oils. Stay out of fast food joints and most restaurants–find a local healthy/organic one and frequent it. You are also going to have to get off of sugar/high-fructose corn syrup entirely, but you can get and use some organic, raw honey and/or pure stevia if you must have something sweet or for use in baking. You can even find sweet things in the health food store that are certified organic like candy bars, licorice, cake mixes, etc. Getting off the GE/glyphosate is the main thing, but as a wonderful side benefit you will be eating many more whole foods that are fundamentally healthier. Put another way, you are simultaneously stopping the bad and starting the good.

Now we have covered what not to eat in the last chapter and what you can eat instead in this chapter. Between the two you can begin what is the first, middle, and ongoing step in my program and turn your gluten thing and general health around–pointed in the right direction now, all you have to do is to keep walking and chugging along. Now you've got that gut issue to deal with, so let's now look at the specific steps in order and cover the details you will need to know to follow them.

Chapter 11: Cleanse the Gut

In terms of considering the order things should be done in, I realized that the gut needs to be cleansed first. Many of the other steps that follow relate to what I was going to take as supplements or eat. I realized that most of these wouldn't be absorbed until and unless the gut was cleaned out.

Imagine that your small intestine is like a water pipe that has gotten all covered in grime, deposits, and sludge around the inside. While the water (food) still flows through the middle (lumen), it can't get to the edges of the pipe (endothelium and villi) where it can be absorbed and used by the body. So, we need something like one of those pipe-cleaning "snakes" that you put in and twist around to clean up the sides of the pipe (small intestine). We also need a way to flush the gunk out as well. Since this gunk or sludge contains nasty stuff and toxins (including glyphosate), it would also be good to have something to soak it up so that it doesn't make us sick after it gets dislodged.

This pipe-cleaning snake is well known: fiber. Think of it like eating sandpaper that scrapes the gunk off of your small intestine and also large intestine (colon) as well. To flush it out we can use anything that acts as a laxative–something that makes you poop fast and frequently. For the sponge, there is this wonderful little plant called Milk Thistle that has the ability and propensity to soak up nasty stuff and then it is carried all the way out in the normal way; It has glutathyamine in it that does this, which also helps it fight or prevent cancer. So does the Azomite listed below in my preferred cleanse; It also has all the minerals you need and this is important because the magnesium oxide you will take tends to strip you of minerals.

So, that's the basic idea and components of a gut cleanse. There are many different types, formulas, and ways to do a gut cleanse. If you already know and have on you like, then feel free to use that one. Or, you can research them and choose from many. But, a word of caution: If you search for "cleanse" or "gut cleanse" on the internet you will find products sold for $50-$300 that are a pure waste of money–you can make your own in less than 5 mins. So, I will provide one in particular because it is very simple, easy, and ridiculously cheap–as in about $15 of supplies will last you a year doing it once a month as a regular monthly maintenance plan. I found out about this cleanse from Shane Ellison, "The People's Chemist", whom I respect a great deal.

Ingredients: 1 or 2 glasses of water, 1 Tbsp Castor Oil, 1 Tbsp Psyllium Husk (men) or 1 heaping tsp (small women), 1 Tbsp Lemon Juice, 500 mg / 50 lbs Magnesium OXIDE (do not use any other form/type), 1 recommended dose Milk Thistle, 1 tsp Azomite.

Note: all of these ingredients are easy to find at a health food store except the Azomite, which is a bit hard to find but Amazon sells it. Your Castor oil is going to last a long time, so keep it refrigerated. Buy a bag of the psyllium husks about the size of a bag of coffee (about a pint)–they often sell it in bulk where you scoop out your own bag. It is typical for magnesium oxide pills to be in 500 mg size. I got it in powder form and your bottle should indicate the milligrams in terms of teaspoons–mine says 1/4 tsp = 700 mg. Don't buy a large amount of this form of magnesium because you want to use a different type for a regular supplement. If you do not find or skip the Azomite, you can substitute a "trace minerals" supplement or a tablespoon of brewer's yeast that are commonly sold in health food stores as well.

Speaking of brewer's yeast, I've used this stuff for years after seeing it listed as a major source of nearly every vitamin. It is also a great source for some folate, selenium, chromium, and also covers all of your essential amino acids–for what you get and how little you use it is also a great bargain. It is commonly made from a bi-product of beer manufacturing, which means it is grown on/with barley. This means it can include tiny amounts of gluten. However, this very tiny amount is only significant for a Celiac person and so I would exclude it being a significant source for when you are going "gluten free" in the 60 day program because you are just using it during the gut cleanse. After the program, since gluten is back on the menu, I highly recommend brewer's yeast on a regular basis as a wonderful supplement and source of key nutrients. I take a tablespoon every single day and have for years.

Also, before rushing to the health food store to buy these gut cleanse ingredients, first read the rest of the book to find some other things you will need as well so you can make one trip. In the summary of steps, a shopping list is included to help you out with this.

Directions: Basically just get the stuff in your body; There are a variety of ways, combinations, and order–and it really doesn't matter how you do it. For example, if your Magnesium is in pill form you can swallow it with the lemon and psyllium water, but if it is in powder you will stir it into the water. The milk thistle will be in a vegicap pill you will swallow. The castor oil won't mix with the water, so you need to take it separately in a big spoon. You can also make one glass filled with the lemon and magnesium, and another with the psyllium and azomite. Or, you can combine it all in one glass. Now I will warn you the castor oil tastes horrid. So, what I do is mix everything into one glass, take the castor oil directly out of a big spoon in one quick gulp and immediately start drinking the mixture in the glass, which gets the taste out fast. It's sort of like chasing a shot of cheap tequila with a beer back.

Further Considerations: The combination of the magnesium oxide and castor oil is a powerful force that is likely to send you nearly rushing to the bathroom to take a #2. I don't mean rushing right after you drink it, but I mean when you feel the urge you don't have a lot of time to make the trip. This is exactly what we are after to "flush" your system. However, this is also going to occur multiple times after you take the cleanse. So, depending upon your job (if you work), you may want to do your cleanse on a day off work. It is best to do the cleanse on a day you can stay at home and always be close to the bathroom. You should also do it on an empty stomach and in the morning. This accomplishes two things: you aren't going to eat the rest of the day and instead begin a short fast, which is our next step; you avoid an "emergency" in the middle of the night while trying to sleep. It is very likely you will have some level of diarrhea, and this is fine. Due to this diarrhea and also needing to encourage a good flush, it is critically important to drink lots of water all day at regular intervals; Continue drinking more water the next day. Since you will be fasting, this will also help alleviate hunger.

Chapter 12: Give your Gut a Break!

Okay, now we have flushed out and cleaned our pipes. Next we want to give our small intestine and entire digestive system a much needed break, some rest, and time to start healing. So, we are going to "fast", or not eat for a while.

Some people may not be good candidates for fasting and it is not appropriate for all people. It may not be healthy to fast–or to fast for very long–if you have a very low body weight or body fat percentage, have anorexia or other eating disorder, high blood pressure, heart problems, or other conditions. You should consult your doctor prior to fasting if any of these apply to you, you have any reasons for concern, and as a general practice. For anyone else it is a good general practice to occasionally do a short period of fasting.

Fasting not only give your system a time out, it will also cause your body to produce more white blood cells, which are a key part of your healing system (immune system). With a replenished army of these little soldiers in your blood, they can help in the battle for the liberty of your gut and you overall health as well. From what I've read, it can take perhaps 3 or 4 days for this effect to kick in. If you can do a 3-4 day fast that would probably be ideal to benefit from this consequence. Longer than that won't give any benefits and you run the risk of depleting yourself of a number of vital nutrients such that it may even be unbeneficial–perhaps even harmful. However, if you lack the will power or other reasons make that too long of a fast, you need to at least fast 1 more full day added on top of yesterday's fast during the gut cleanse. So, you will be doing at least a 2-day fast in total.

Speaking of needing nutrients, we know how important amino acids are and that we don't store them–we need them daily. Two days without them isn't going to cause a major issue, but it is still wise to get some. Also, if you are doing a 3-4 day fast it becomes even more important to get your amino acids. Now then, since we can't eat, it seems impossible to get our amino acids (protein). However, they make a great product called "Bragg's Amino Acids" that you can get at the health food store. It is in liquid form. So, you can add the amount suggested on the bottle to one of the glasses of water you are drinking. Since they are the core amino acids in simple form and not a complex protein, no digestion is required and we are thus still giving our digestive system a rest.

A fast is pretty simple and easy: don't eat any food. Other than that there are some things we can discuss about what you drink. What we are after is mostly a "water fast", which means you aren't drinking juices, beer, wine, fruit smoothies, etc. If you are like me, it's fine if you can't skip your morning coffee, but don't drink anything else except water and perhaps some tea.

With your water it is a good idea to keep adding some lemon juice, but just add to taste and not as much as you did for the cleanse. If you want, you can add a little honey as well. This will help give you some energy and the sugars get into your system very fast without much real digestive work occurring. But, don't use sugar because it is made from GMO sugar beets and you are going "glyphosate free"–as previously discussed.

If you are a tea drinker that's great and drink whatever you like. However, black tea is a great one for this time because it acts as a "pre-biotic" that is going to help your probiotics, which will be our next step. Black tea is also an antioxidant. Of course it has a bit of caffeine that might help your energy level if you are feeling tired from not eating.

Another thing/tea you can drink that would be good right now is a ginger tea because ginger is well known to calm the stomach, help the stomach, and also to kills viruses, bacteria, etc. You can begin drinking this on Day 1, which is your cleanse day. You can see how the black tea and ginger tea are going to help a bit with what we are trying to accomplish. You can buy some ginger tea packages, or you can just buy raw ginger root and make your own. I recommend this because it is cheaper, raw ginger is better, and you can also eat it after meals once your fast is over. Just slice up a half inch or so very thin and boil it in a pan of water for 15 minutes. Strain that and add some lemon and honey to make your tea. You will have several glasses of tea to use during the day or evening.

After you are done with your fast there are a few things to consider. If you only did a short fast, the first one isn't that big of a deal. However, if you fasted 3 or 4 days then you might want to ease back into eating. You will want to start with small portions of things that are easy to digest. Consider "comfort foods" and things that are cooked, soft, and carbohydrates like potatoes or bread. Obviously the bread would have to be both gluten free and also organic. Soups are a good idea as well. Some things to avoid or take slowly would be things hard to digest such as raw vegetable and red meat. Just take things a bit slow and easy the first day or two after a longer fast–don't pig out just because you can eat again!

Pretty soon after your short fast, or easing back in from a longer one, it would be a good idea to now focus on eating a few more cooked vegetables, beans, oatmeal, nuts, seeds, and other grains. The reason you want to do this is because of their high fiber content. This will serve to do a bit more of the gut cleanse just like the psyllium did. So, eat plenty of fiber for the next several days after you break your fast. By the end of this your small and large intestines should be well cleaned out. Don't jump right into the raw vegetables or eat too many of them at this point. The reason for this is you don't have a healthy gut flora colony to digest them yet and they are harder to digest generally when raw because cooking them helps break apart the cellulose structure. In the next step we will build that colony of gut flora up and then you can go for it on lots of fresh, raw veggies.

<u>Review:</u> Fast for at least one more day after your gut cleanse; fast for another day or two if you can; During your fast just drink liquids such as water, water with lemon juice, tea, black tea, and ginger tea (add a little honey to teas if you want); Add Bragg's Amino Acids to your water. Break a long fast by easing in to it with small portions and easy to digest foods. Then start eating some fiber, but don't overdue it on vegetables–in particular raw ones.

Another big part of "giving your gut a break" relates to giving your villi a break as well as giving your gut a break from trying to deal with gluten/gliadin. Let's talk about that next.

Chapter 13: Spare your Villi

Some of the steps in my program overlap each other, so keep this in mind as you implement it. This "step" is a case in point. Beginning at this point you are going to want to eliminate from your diet a few other foods even though they aren't necessarily GE ones.

I'm sure you were paying attention, have a perfect memory, and recall there were four food types that harm your villi: Corn, soy, wheat, and casein. Until you complete this 2-month program, do not eat these foods either. The reason should be obvious: you are healing your gut and your villi are a major part that these foods damage. So, spare your villi by taking a break from these.

Corn should be easy enough to avoid, but just consider you are going to need to read labels and avoid things like the corn meal, corn starch, as well as things like corn chips, corn-based cereals, corn tortillas, etc. High-fructose corn syrup is something else you cannot consume, but any form of sugar should already be off your list as it all is GE/glyphosate, is fundamentally unhealthy, and feeds candida as well–so it goes against the work you will do to rebuild your colony of probiotics/gut flora. Later on you can eat some of these foods as long as they are organic.

Soy is pretty much all genetically engineered. Besides that, it is generally unhealthy and messing up your hormones. Therefore, you should just stop eating soy for the rest of your life. Anyone who thinks soy is wonderful and is all into tofu and soy protein powders simply doesn't have the facts/science in my opinion–ignore them or what you might believe about soy as it isn't good stuff. Just consider that eating raw soy is poisonous; That alone should tell you something; It is as if the "Creator" itself said, "Don't eat this!" All combined, this means not eating mainly soy products such as soymilk, tofu, etc. But it also means watching out for and not eating the soy lecithin they put/sneak into dang near every processed food that we discussed earlier.

Wheat is not a GE crop, but it is going to be off your diet for about 6 weeks for two good reasons: the damaging effect on your villi; giving your gut a break from the gliadin until it is repaired enough to be able to handle it. Basically we are healing the gut and don't want to be pissing it off and causing inflammation in the meantime, which is contrary to healing. After your gut is healed, there will be a step in the program to slowly re-introduce wheat; By that time you should be able to digest the gliadin with your healthy colony of gut flora and your villi will be repaired and strong enough to handle some. Even so, you will have to only eat organic wheat due to the glyphosate residue issue.

So just for a while during the healing process, you are going to be going "gluten free" if you haven't done so already.

Personally what I did was to find a great wheat and gluten free bread recipe online and made my own bread. It was a simple recipe, the bread was great, and it didn't require a bread maker. It Isn't enough to try to get gluten free bread at this point because it still has wheat in it–they just remove the gluten. So the issue is that type of bread would still hurt your villi that you are trying to give a break. For the bread I made, I used brown rice flour.

In terms of going gluten free, it is important to realize that wheat isn't the only source of gluten/gliadin. Barley is another grain with gliadin in it. While you may not be eating barley in a bowl, you may be drinking it. Barley is a big ingredient in beer. If you drink beer, you need to either stop doing it for 6 weeks or you can find and buy gluten free beer. Distilled alcohols can't have gluten in them as already mentioned, so if you want to drink alcohol, you can switch to wine or "the hard stuff". Just be aware you can't use mixes such as sodas made with the high-fructose corn syrup. However, you can find organic sodas or mixers.

There are also other wheat types and derivatives to avoid that contain gliadin: wheat berries, durum, emmer, semolina, spelt, farina, farro, graham, kamut/khorasan wheat, and einkorn wheat. Other grains that include gluten/gliadin aren't commonly eating, but they include these: malt, bulgur, rye, seitan, triticale and mir (a cross between wheat and rye). My mom used to make us bulgur, bless her heart, but the stuff should have been called "vulgar" instead and I can't fathom who would willingly eat that crud. But if you are a vulgar eater, knock it off for now.

Now the casein you are going to cut out for 6 weeks as well. Casein is a protein found in milk, and of course products made from it such as cream, sour cream, and cheese. It is notoriously hard to digest casein, and thus hard on the villi. Some people are even allergic to it.

I've read that once a person has gluten intolerance their body can develop intolerance to other proteins because it basically mistakes them for gluten/gliadin. In a way, they are too similar for it to differentiate, or perhaps the body decides that since it is so dang hard to digest it must be that darn gliadin. I don't know if this is true, or if those are proper explanations, but I do have some personal experience that tends to confirm it.

When I first went gluten free I found that milk, cheese, and even eggs seemed to produce symptoms. When I researched this I found out that basically the body has generalized or mistaken these proteins and thus created something like a cross-allergic reaction. Because we want to minimize any inflammation so our guts can heal, we are also going to take a 1-month break from casein and eggs. So, this means no milk, things with milk in them, cream, 1/2 and 1/2, cheese, cream cheese, sour cream, or foods/products with cheese in them such as Cheetos, Doritos, cheese crackers, mac-n-cheese, etc. Notice that those processed foods just mentioned have corn or wheat in them anyway.

The same goes for eggs in terms of perhaps having a mistaken/similar protein, but I don't think they are as much of an issue. Take at least a 2 week break from eggs; Then try them and see if you have any reactions or not. If you do, stay off them for the 4 weeks, if not then you can eat them occasionally during this period. Personally I think eggs are one of the near-perfect foods. Consider that an egg has everything required for tiny embryo to develop into a chick! The only supposed negative about eggs is the cholesterol, which is actually a non-issue because cholesterol is very healthy and there is no causal relationship between it and heart issues–it is more about the fibrinogen, which they don't gave a pill for and thus ignore, but that is a whole other long story. The bottom line is that eggs are wonderful for you as well as the other foodstuffs that contain all things required for life: brewer's yeast, blue-green algae, and chlorella (fresh-water algae). And fry them in real, organic butter–it is a great source of healthy fat and ignore anyone who says otherwise!

This part about casein and eggs isn't as critically important as the other aspect of the program. But, please do you best to not eat these things. If you simply can't or won't, then at least eat as little as possible, and also try to go completely off of them for a least some period of time. After that you can slowly re-introduce them–that will be covered later along with reintroducing corn and even wheat. Also, as was mentioned with the eggs, if you do have a little bit of casein, see how your body responds and if it complains then stay off it for 4 weeks.

Summary and Review: To spare your villi and give them time to heal, you are going to stop eating corn, soy, wheat, other gliadin grains like barley, and casein products immediately following your fast. You will do this for corn and casein for about a month, wheat for 6 weeks, and soy forever. You will also not eat eggs for about a month because they may sort of be mistaken for gluten or your body has developed something like a cross-allergy to them and casein. Do your best with this, and you can test out eggs after two weeks. At this point in the program you also aren't eating any GM/glyphosate foods outright, nor any foods or products that have GE ingredients.

Chapter 14: Rebuilding your Colony

We are now turning towards the part of the solution that has to do with rebuilding our colony of gut flora (healthy bacteria or probiotics). The sooner we get a bunch of these wonderful friends and assistants doing their jobs to help us out the better. So, there is no sense in wasting any time.

I think it would be pointless to start taking probiotics on the first day of the program because the cleanse is going to cause everything to move through and out your system really fast–perhaps even "shoot" out of your system. You could potentially start taking probiotics the day afterwards, but this depends upon how your system is dealing with the cleanse. In other words, you may still be doing some flushing and might, for example, still have a little diarrhea. If so, you definitely want to wait another day to begin. Even if you don't, it might still be a good idea to wait until day 3 or after you break your fast to begin. Why might this be?

Well, keep in mind these probiotics are living organisms and they need to eat to survive. We also know these gut flora are going to need some magnesium and sulfur as well. Since we will next move into repair/regenerate stage, your intestinal walls and villi will need those as well. So, let's begin doing some probiotics and also these minerals after we break the fast to ensure they live.

Taking the probiotics is simple and straightforward in general. But, there are many products and some details to consider. Firstly, off-the-shelf probiotics come in two forms: capsules or liquids. Both can be found at a health food store. Because they are alive and won't benefit you if they are dead, they are refrigerated which sort of puts them in hibernation and ensures they don't cook to death. So ask for help in the store locating them. That was especially true in the past; However, they now have freeze-dried and powdered forms that apparently do not require refrigeration.

If what you get does need to be refrigerated (or kept cool and dry) then consider that when shopping: for example you might want to take a small cooler, shop in the morning, and definitely don't go make another shopping trip and leave them in a hot car in summer. They will likely say on the bottle to ensure stored below 72 degrees Fahrenheit, but you should refrigerate them at home regardless.

Let's take what they call "kefir culture starters" first. So the health food stores sell these small bottles (usually 4, 8 or 16 ozs) of liquid that have billions of the bacteria in them. People usually use these to make kefirs of many sorts, ferment vegetables, make yogurt, etc. It is like getting a package of yeast to make bread. Once you put the yeast in warm water it starts to reproduce, and these little guys do that very fast and at an exponential rate. So, you can take a small portion of this kefir starter and use it to make big batches of stuff.

However, you can also simply drink the kefir starter and have them take up residence directly in your gut and start their orgy and reproductive spree right there. The benefit of doing this is that you get a massive amount of them compared to taking capsules of probiotics. You don't necessarily have to drink the whole bottle. What I have done is to get an 8 oz bottle of kefir starter and drank half of it one day and half the next. I think it is a good way to get a good jump-start going for building your colony.

This brings up the general point that it is likely best to do what amounts to a massive first intake of probiotics. What this does is get a big enough colony going that enough survive and can reproduce. Stomach acid may kill some or perhaps some don't find a nice home in your intestinal walls and end up literally being flushed. After a big initial dose or several, then you can take a daily "maintenance" dosage to keep a nice fresh supply and ensure your colony is large, strong, and continues to flourish.

The other form and option you have is the capsules. In the health food store you will likely find many options and not know which to purchase. It is probably a good idea to ask for help to find time locating them and finding a good one; They too are usually refrigerated.

What are good probiotics to choose? First of all there are many strains/species of these bacteria. They are all "good" and likely none is "superior" to the others. In general what you want is a diverse colony in your gut that has quite a few strains. You want multiple strains because they each do you some slightly different services; They have certain specialties and preferences for what they want to break down. So the bottom line is that you want to find a probiotics supplement that has multiple strains in it. You want at least 3 or 4 I would think if they are the primary and best known to be helpful strains. Even so, the general rule is the more the merrier and a half dozen or more strains would be ideal.

Second of all, an important thing to consider is that these things are microscopic. So you literally have to take billions of them to amount to being beneficial, or even close to the shear numbers that will eventually inhabit your colony. Their numbers are so vast that these guys actually outnumber all the rest of the cells in your body combined! So in general you want "a big number" on the bottle. You might find a bottle on the shelf that says, "5 billion live probiotics" and be impressed and temped to buy it, but that is likely a less expensive product and not near what you really want–or you will simply have to take more of the capsules.

What you are looking for is to find one that has at least 20 billion, and there are certainly ones with 40, 50, 80 billion, or more. The price usually goes up as the count does, but you can do a little rough Math to find the right balance. For example, if the 80 billion costs more than twice the 40 billion then it would be cheaper to buy the 40's and just take more of them; If it is less expensive, then get the higher count.

Personally I've been using a Vitacost brand that has 20 billion (2 capsule serving size) and 10 different strains. By the way, I do a lot of shopping from the online retailer Vitacost because they have fantastic prices, discounts, free shipping for quantity orders, and a massive inventory of products; They are sort of the Amazon for health related products. If you don't live close to a health food store, consider using Vitacost to get your supplies for this program and for your other needs. No, they don't pay me for plugging them, but they should!

So I would suggest you tell the person at the store you are looking for probiotic capsules (and/or go check out the kefir starters), and once you get there tell them you are looking for one that has at least 20 billion and want one with quite a few strains. See what they suggest, compare a few for quantity, strain count, and price. I would also suggest that if you end up getting one with only a single strain or just a few strains that you save the bottle and also keep a log of what strains you took. When you need to buy another bottle, select a different brand and get one with different strains. By doing this you will help build a more diverse colony.

For my program what you are going to do is hit the probiotics in big doses for 2 or 3 days. When I started my program–or when I ran out or slacked off taking them–I take 80 billion per day in a single dose on an empty stomach in the morning (after my coffee). You could also split the dose and do the other half before bed–hopefully you aren't eating close to bedtime and again have an empty stomach. I would consider the half bottle of kefir starter about the same, but read the bottle you purchase. After that initial start-up dose, keep taking your probiotics daily at the dosage level indicated on the bottle.

I personally don't think they are very expensive, so I just pop the capsules. But, if you find them cost-prohibitive then you can easily find out how to make your own kefirs, fermented foods, yogurt, etc via the internet, books, or by checking with friends. Some of these would then be things you would drink; Others you would eat and incorporate into meals. Just to give you an idea of cost savings, that one bottle of kefir culture starter would likely last you a year to make your own fermented foods–and it is perhaps the same price as a month's supply of capsules. However, these things take some education, time, purchasing foodstuffs in many cases, and some require regular maintenance and tending. Since learning how to make these takes time, just use the capsules (or just drink the kefir starter) during my program so you can get going with it; You can then learn and make your own kefirs and fermented foods later if you wish to continue your daily maintenance dose of probiotics using them, or you can use the supplement form.

<u>Summary and Review:</u> Put probiotics on your shopping list, buy some that have a large number count and multiple strains; keep them cool; start taking probiotics the next day after you complete your fast. Take about 80 billion count of the capsules for 3 days in the morning on an empty stomach, or divide that dosage in two and take morning/night. Alternatively drink about 4 ozs of kefir starter each day for 2 to 3 days and then use capsules or a smaller quantity of starter. After this initial high start-up dosage, continue to take the dosage indicated on your product daily–not just for the rest of the program, but for the rest of your life! After you get your colony beefed up, you can eat more vegetables including raw ones to do some more good cleansing of your intestines.

Chapter 15: Supplement your Healing and Health

As per the general strategy, we now turn to the phase of my program where you will be focusing on healing or repairing your gut in terms of the physical and cellular structures. Once again this step overlaps a bit with the previous ones. So, you can begin the actions of this step as soon as you break your fast; It overlaps with building up your colony of gut flora.

Most of this phase of the program extends the entire 2 months as it entails what is required to support your gut healing itself by supplying it the nutrients it needs. However, many of the supplements and dietary suggestions apply well after the program because they are also key things required to maintain your gut and overall health.

Gathered from our previous discussions and adding a few new items, here is a list of the supplements or nutrients that will support the healing process and time period your gut is making physical repairs; These also include things glyphosate is probably depleting or negatively impacting:

Supplements and Nutrients for Healing: amino acids, magnesium, sulfur, ginger root, black tea, probiotics, healthy whole foods, and milk thistle. New items: real/raw vitamin supplements, garlic, sodium bicarbonate, folate, and turmeric extract.

Let's work our way through this list so you know why these will help, what/how to get them, and what to put on your shopping list. We have already sufficiently discussed the ginger root tea, black tea, probiotics, and milk thistle. I include them here so you have a complete list. Just continue to use them during this phase of the program. Continue to take a serving of milk thistle daily; It is a great way to keep flushing out any food or environmental toxins as well as remove cellular waste and oxidation that is generally unhealthy and can contribute to cancer.

In terms of healthy whole foods we can have a fairly brief discussion so you understand how they will benefit your gut healing and overall health. Certainly there are entire books devoted to this topic. Remember that all your body's systems are inter-connected and inter-dependant; Also, recall that glyphosate has likely messed up other organs and system such as your liver, kidney, hormones, enzymes, and neurotransmitters, etc.

In general there is a key benefit to eating whole foods because it seems nature has included in a food certain things required to digest and utilize what is in them. The body cannot use many vitamins independently; They require other vitamins as "synergists". At times, other things such as a key mineral are required for absorption and utilization (often the term "bio-available" is used to partially describe this).

A citric fruit or other vitamin C rich food is a good example of this principle. Typically vitamin C is called "ascorbic acid", but that is only one part of what comes in the whole food that our body requires to make use of it. The full package also includes these: ascorbigen bi-flavanoid complexes, P factors, K factors, J factors, and tyrosinase. All of these are actually required for the vitamin C to become bio-available and utilized by the body–work needs to be done on the ascorbic acid in the liver first and it needs these synergists.

There are numerous cases similar to this. As a general example, many of the B vitamins require other B vitamins in order to carry out certain functions, and the foods that contain one of these often have the others. Another example would be that you cannot utilize iron without having B12, but we find the best sources for iron, such as liver and other meats, are also the best sources of B12. I nearly seems like there is some intelligence or planning behind what makes up the foods that nature makes because most of them appear to be this "complete package" where all the synergists are included to ensure bioavailability and performance of key functions in our bodies. We are about to discuss magnesium, and magnesium absorption is increased by, or requires, protein (amino acids). Would you guess that many whole foods high in magnesium just so happen to also be high in protein?

In summary then, eating whole foods helps ensure we get all that we need to make use of the various nutrients. Whole foods give us nature's well designed "complete package". Eating much more of these complete packages will provide our gut and body more of what they need to repair and maintain themselves.

In contrast, refined and processed foods are only including a portion of the original whole package. Consider something like corn. It is likely impossible to get too much sugar from eating whole corn–imagine trying to eat a bushel of it in one sitting; But if you take an entire bushel and extract just the sugars as high-fructose corn syrup, then you can consume the bushel in one soda pop; You won't be getting all the fiber, oil, vitamins, and proteins that would have helped your body process the fructose in a healthy way, timeframe, and amount. So two major issues with processed foods are that they extract and compress things, and they also then omit other important required nutrients and synergists.

Since Americans are very deficient in magnesium and also eat lots of processed foods, you have to wonder if that deficiency is partially due to not eating enough whole foods that have that magnesium in them. For example, only one of the top 10 foods containing the highest levels of magnesium can be found in a cheeseburger or pizza; That one is actually grains, but the whole grain has more magnesium than just the flour made from it–nature intended that we eat the entire grain. So the cheeseburger or pizza doesn't really have whole grain anyway. Most of the dense protein is found in the outer germ and bran portions of the grain–normally the discarded "chaff" that is taken out prior to making flour. The benefit of the whole grain is so well known that it is why you see labels such as "whole grain bread", or "whole grain cereal", or "with whole grains".

Since that top 10 list came up, let's include it now so that you have a good list of whole foods to focus on to beef up your magnesium intake by eating whole foods. Also consider that since we know all life forms require and use magnesium, there is some amount in any whole food you consume. The following list is basically ranked in order from the highest magnesium content to lowest, but they are all wonderful sources. **For the next two months focus on eating a lot of these as whole foods rich in Magnesium** (except the yogurt due to casein, but after the program it is fine and be sure to get it "with live cultures", which are probiotics–but many brands are very high in sugar or use high-fructose corn syrup). Note: I have deleted barley and bulgur from the list due to them containing gluten:

DARK LEAFY GREENS (1 cup and % Daily Value): Spinach (39%), Swiss Chard (38%), Kale (19%), Collard Greens (13%), and Turnip Greens (11%). **SEEDS** (1 oz handful or 28 grams): Squash/Pumpkin Seeds (39%), Hemp Seeds (50%), Flax (28%), Sesame (25%), Chia (24%), and Sunflower Seeds (9%). **BEANS AND LENTILS** (1 cup or 170 grams): Lima Beans (31%), White Beans (28%), French Beans (25%), Black-eyed Peas (23%), Kidney Beans (21%), Chickpeas/Garbanzos (20%), Lentils (18%), and Pinto Beans (16%). **WHOLE GRAINS** (1 cup or 195 grams): Brown Rice (21%), Quinoa (30%), Millet (19%), Buckwheat (13%), Wild Rice (13%), and Oats (7%). **FISH** (3oz fillet): Mackerel (21%), Pollock (18%), Turbot (14%), Tuna (14%), Wild Trout (13%), and Cod (9%). **NUTS** (1oz handful or 28 grams): Almonds (20%), Brazilnuts (27%), Cashews (18%), Pine Nuts (18%), Hazelnuts (12%), Walnuts (11%), and Pecans (9%). **Dark Chocolate/85% Cocoa** 1oz square or 28g (16%). **YOGURT** 1 cup or 245 grams (12%). **AVOCADO** 1 cup cubed or 150 grams (11%). **BANANAS** 1 medium or 118 grams (8%).

Many other vegetables are high in magnesium as well. Here are some notable mentions with high levels: **squash, artichoke, peas, okra, and potatoes.**

Just for a moment, consider how healthy a robust salad would be if you include things from the above list. I happen to love beans in my salad–in particular garbanzo and kidney beans. If you haven't tried beans in your salads then do so. Considering the above list, just imagine how much magnesium, potassium, vitamins, etc. you would be eating in this salad: spinach, (and maybe some kale or turnip greens), beans, sunflower seeds, sliced raw almonds, mushrooms, and half an avocado. You could make your own healthy dressing with sunflower oil and lemon juice (or vinegar). After a month when you can eat casein again, you can also make a good salad dressing based upon plain yogurt, which won't have the sugar and also has the probiotics. Also at that time you could add in a sliced hard-boiled egg.

Basically, most fruits are pretty high in magnesium, but we want to avoid them for a while or just eat a little because we don't want to feed the unhealthy gut parasite candida. I use a frozen banana in my morning protein shake for taste, to make it like a milkshake, and because they are also high in the important mineral potassium. Since I brought it up, I actually spent 6 months researching nutrients that led me to create a shake that contains basically all your nutrients. All of the information, ingredients, and details of how to make it are in my book, "Total Health thru Complete Nutrition: Matt's Marvelous Shake." Getting that book and making Matt's shake would go a long way towards you being able to quickly and easily get all of your nutrients, which would go a long way in supporting the process of healing your gut, other ailments and issues, and improving your overall health. A key benefit of my shake is that it is much simpler and faster than trying to shop and prepare the wide variety of whole foods that would be needed to provide the same complete nutrient profile. If you are a busy person, or just not that into vegetables and/or cooking, it may be a very valuable book and shake program for you.

Let's get back to the above list. Most of the above foods are also very high in potassium such as fish, beans, avocados, potatoes, squash, and yogurt. So eating these will give you both magnesium and potassium. Mushrooms are very healthy in multiple ways and also have lots of magnesium and potassium.

We should all know that generally speaking vegetables, seeds, nuts, fish, etc. are healthy. They contain more wonderful and health-promoting things than we can cover in this book. But suffice it to say that when you eat lots of whole foods you will be getting tons of vitamins, bio-flavanoids, vitamins, minerals, protein, healthy fats/oils, complex carbohydrates, amino acids, fiber, etc. So, eating the whole foods not only helps us get the magnesium that is so critical to repairing our gut and feeding our flora, but eating whole foods also provides many other required nutrients they need–including the key ones required to be able to make new cells; On top of that, all of these are very helpful and healing to our entire body as well.

Look again at the list and notice that beans, nuts, seeds, fish, and even grains are all good sources of protein; Remember that protein is a synergist for magnesium. In addition, potassium and magnesium are synergists and work together for many body functions. Some of these foods are good sources for folate and also B12–both of these plus magnesium are required to make a new cell, which your body does millions of times each day. So once again we see the "complete package" principle of nature and whole foods.

Speaking of new cells, which I have mentioned several times, we are in the phase of repairing and rebuilding the cells that make up our villi and the walls/lining of our intestine as well.

To make a new cell these things are required: magnesium, folate, B12, and amino acids.

We have just covered magnesium, so let's explore the rest of this list–which also was in our main list of supplementing our healing anyway.

Folate is an essential nutrient primarily found in plants. "They" are now changing the name to call it "folic acid", but this is a misnomer since they are not the same and there is a man-made and pharmaceutical folic acid that is not the same and very likely not even healthy to consume. So, you want real folate from nature, not the Frankenfolicacid made in chemical laboratories by drug pushers.

What is folate? You may be unfamiliar with that name, but you have likely heard it more commonly referred to as B9. It is water soluble, which means any excess is eliminated in your urine and you can't store it up; So, it is very important to get your folate/B9 daily. Folate primarily helps the body make new cells and in particular works in copying and synthesizing DNA, of which magnesium is also a key part. Folate helps the body utilize vitamin B12 and amino acids. So you can see it is a both the building material for new cells and also one of those required synergists for B12 and amino acids–they need it to do their jobs.

Eating green vegetables as whole foods is going to help you get your folate, and we know things like spinach and other green vegetables are also high in magnesium and potassium. So those are certainly foods to eat a lot of.

To repair your gut and build new cells, be sure to eat lots of folate during this program. While any green vegetable is going to be high in folate, here are some other notable good sources of it: Spinach, asparagus, and broccoli; probably those nasty Brussels sprouts; Beans such as garbanzo beans, pinto beans, and lentils; black-eyed peas, liver, and avocado.

As you can see, meat is not a substantial source, but I guess some is stored or being used in the liver. I suppose if one can stomach that nasty stuff, then there is one good meat/animal source for folate.

Based upon all the nutrients we have been discussing, perhaps our wise older mothers knew best when they told us to eat our vegetables. Or, if your mom was like mine, she insisted you eat them–or you had to stair at peas or Brussels sprouts on your plate for 3 hours at the table until you fell asleep and outlasted her through sheer will and stubbornness!

The bottom line point is: eat your dang vegetables and especially the green ones! You simply must have the folate in them and you need to get it every day!

We want to get the folate and lots of vitamins from our vegetables. However, cooking and high heat kills or destroys these. So, it is best to eat your vegetables raw whenever possible. For ones you are cooking, you want to just "tender cook" or steam them very lightly. I've read things about how cooking a vegetable for 3 minutes kills something like 30% of the vitamins, but even just 2 more minutes kills 70%. So, pay attention when cooking them, test often, and as soon as they are done remove them from heat–if boiling, take them out of the hot water.

Another tip is that if you are making things that are combinations of veggies, soups, stews, etc. then you can time when you add various things. For example, you may need to boil the potatoes for 40 minutes to get them done, but you can add the other veggies basically at the last minute and take your pot off heat as soon as they are done–or even slightly prior as they will continue to cook. Besides saving the vitamins and folate, tender-cooked veggies taste better and don't get all mushy. Some things like celery, onions, etc. can barely be cooked or put in at the very end to be left raw and provide a bit of crunch and texture. Microwave ovens are known to kill/nuke vitamins–don't cook veggies in them or use them to re-heat them.

Important tip: Do not overcook your veggies or you will lose a ton of the folate and vitamins! Do not nuke them in a microwave!! Eat your veggies raw whenever possible!!!

Next on our list is B12, or Cobalamin. This is the largest and most complex of all vitamins and is involved in many important processes. We are focusing on it because of how it works with making new cells and as a synergist to metabolizing and working with amino acids. B12 is sort of the opposite of folate in that it comes almost entirely from meat/animal sources and is almost absent in plants.

Accordingly, B12 deficiency is a common issue for vegans and vegetarians, and it has horrid consequences including mania and even permanent psychological damage–it has a long list of side effects as well. Nearly every source I've read about B12 says that vegan and vegetarians cannot possibly get enough of it and must supplement it. We will discuss vitamin supplementation and a related issue later in this chapter. My book, "Total Health thru Complete Nutrition: Matt's Marvelous Shake" reveals a very specific type of B12 vitamin supplement that is actually plant based and organic that vegans and vegetarians would really benefit from. Additionally, the shake covers all nutrients including amino acids, which are both a challenge for non-meat eaters to get without a ton of knowledge and careful meal planning involving complex calculations.

Most all meat and dairy foods are good sources for B12. Here are some of the top ones: liver, red meat, fish, crab, shellfish, milk, cheese, yogurt, and eggs.

Since you are going to be off of casein (milk/cheese) and eggs for a while, at this stage you are going to have to focus on eating enough meat and fish, or to take a B12 supplement–or injection. I strongly advise against taking the common B12 supplements because nearly all of them are pharmaceutical drugs and not real vitamin B12–again, see my other book for how to get the real stuff.

Also consider that eating enough healthy meats is also going to give you lots of protein, or amino acids, which is the next item on our lists of both supplementing our health and what is required to make new cells. Of course you will want to get organic grass fed beef and other organic meats to avoid glyphosate residue. Note: I personally do not think residue in the meat/muscle is a large issue or significant source–it is much more likely to be an issue in the bones, ligaments, and connective tissues; however, while on the program it would be best to avoid the potential, so for now you should focus on organic meats. When we discuss sulfur you will discover another benefit and reason to eat organic meat.

We've already extensively discussed amino acids and how vital they are to our bodies in tons of ways. We know we need them to make any cell and new tissues. All that leaves to be discussed is to ensure you are getting enough of it each day during your stage of healing and repairing your gut; Remember that you can't store amino acids, so you need to eat them each day.

Of course we can easily get lots of amino acids by eating meats, which is nice because that also gives us our critical B12. Additionally, we know that all those seeds, nuts, beans, and legumes are all good sources for lots of protein. Between eating a lot of those whole foods and eating fish and various meats, you can probably get all the protein you need. You just have to stay conscious of getting enough each day.

Speaking of which, what if you get to the end of the day and realize you didn't get enough (about 50 grams) of your protein? Well, since you bought those Bragg's Amino Acids for your fast, you can also use those to get your amino acids–keep in mind you will be doing a monthly cleanse and fast anyway that strongly suggests you buy and use these, so you can use them to supplement your amino acids since you already have them on hand.

Another option for getting enough protein/amino acids includes drinking a shake/smoothie that has some type of protein powder in it. There are so many protein powders to choose from and finding a good one can be tough and require some knowledge. There are also some "not good" ones and even "very unhealthy" ones out there. It is too much to go into in this book, but naturally I cover this in my other book, "Total Health thru Complete Nutrition: Matt's Marvelous Shake". So, if you want to go the route of protein powder supplementation I strongly encourage you to get that book and make my shake. In my book I reveal a particular great protein powder that is basically "pre-digested", that means it would be ideal to use while you are healing your gut whose digestive capability is impaired right now– in particular in terms of digesting protein. It is also a wise choice for older people who are known to have less digestive enzymes.

In terms of protein, you want to get about 50 grams of protein each day. But, this can vary up/down a little for your body weight. Most protein powders will have you add 1 scoop, which is usually from 20 to 25 grams of protein. As a general rule, one serving of something like meat or beans gives you about half of what you need in a day. To get more precise, you can read labels or use the internet to find out the actual protein content of what you are eating or normally eat.

The U.S. government spent over a decade creating a list/database of all the nutrient profiles of every food–including processed ones and even fast foods. So, you can just enter a search for something like, "How much protein is in (fill in the blank). The results will lead you to any number of websites that are searching the government database. Bookmark one and use it to look up various protein foods for a while until you get a handle on how much of which foods you need to eat to get your daily dose of amino acids. Vegans and vegetarians should really be doing this search and doing the Math for every meal and have daily totals.

With amino acids now covered, we've completed the "making new cells" list and can continue with the rest of the original list of things we need to ensure we are getting.

In summary, between eating red meat, poultry, fish, nuts/seeds, and beans you can get a lot of protein; You can also combine this with a daily protein shake; Alternatively you can either normally or on an as-needed basis use Bragg's Amino Acids. After 6 weeks on the program, you can also add back eggs, yogurt, and cheese to your diet as other good sources of protein.

We found that glyphosate blocks sulfur pathways and that sulfur is a very important. Therefore, we want to ensure that we are getting enough of it. Sulfur is a mineral and is present in every single cell in your body. Sulfur is critical for your liver to be able to detoxify; If glyphosate is a toxic substance that is getting inside our body, hopefully our liver is trying to get it out–but it will require sulfur to get the job done. Some of the healthiest cultures in the world just so happen to have the highest levels of sulfur in their diet; The U.S. has one of the lowest levels and you know its health is in the toilet.

The first source of sulfur I want to mention is garlic. Garlic is well known to be very healthy and in particular is good for healing a multitude of bacteria and viruses–including ones for which there are no medications or antibiotics. Garlic has been used for health reasons for thousands of years. But, what is in the garlic that is so darn good for our bodies?

As it turns out, garlic has tons of sulfoaphane in it. Sulfoaphane is easily converted by the body into a usable form of sulfur. So really it is the sulfur providing many of the benefits, and garlic provides it in a wonderful form. Some people object to eating a lot of garlic due to the offensive affect on the breath. Mouthwash is a potential solution for that, but if you eat a ton of garlic it won't completely deal with the issue. However, they also now have "odorless garlic extract" capsules that you can take as a supplement. In addition to being odorless, they are incredibly inexpensive. Garlic is also known to reduce blood pressure and is good for the heart and circulatory system. So, consider eating lots of garlic or taking it as an odorless supplement to get more sulfur.

The next good idea is somewhat of an old folk medicine and remedy for tons of ailments and conditions: Epsom salt. Most commonly it is used to take a salt bath by adding 2 cups of it to your bath water (sometimes combined with regular salt or baking soda). You then soak for at least 15 minutes in it; Do not add any soap, or at least not during the soak. You can also add 1/2 cup to a basin of warm water and soak your feet in it, which helps them feel better after a long day and isn't as much of a task as taking the full bath.

While it is called "salt" due to its structure, it isn't really a salt and doesn't have any sodium in it. What is in it are two things: Magnesium and Sulfur! It is Magnesium Sulfate, or MgSO4 chemically. Since we want both magnesium and sulfur to heal and build up our gut/cells/bodies, then Epsom salt seems a great source—it is just the two put together in one cheap and widely available form.

When Epsom salt is dissolved in water, the magnesium and sulfur/sulfate are broken apart. For a bath, the theory is that these are then absorbed through the skin. Some say they cannot be absorbed through the skin, yet others claim there are multiple studies showing they can be absorbed. Based upon hundreds of years of people taking Epsom salt baths, it seems it does get absorbed and helps with inflammation, tired muscles, arthritis, constipation, and many other ailments.

Regardless, Epsom salt can also be taken orally. Just dissolve about 1/2 teaspoon in a glass of water and drink it. This would be about 350-400 mg each of sulfur and magnesium. The RDA for magnesium is set by age and gender: Males 19-30 yrs. 400 mg and 420 mg over 30; Females 19-30 yrs. 310 mg and 320 mg over 30. Therefore, for a male the 1/2 tsp is about right and a female can do a tad less or use 3/8 tsp if you have one or 3 measure of 1/8 tsp.

Most sources I've checked say that magnesium is well tolerated and getting too much isn't really an issue since the body will simply not absorb it; The main thing of getting too much might be some slight stomach upset and diarrhea. So, try these dosages and if those happen then back off the amount slightly until you tolerate it well. You can also consider how much you are getting from food and adjust it accordingly. On days you know that you are not, or did not, eating a lot of magnesium rich foods you can do the full dose. But if you are going for the list of magnesium rich foods, then perhaps cut the dose by half. If you don't know, take a half dose in the morning and then take the other half in the evening only if needed.

Keep in mind the RDA levels are set for "healthy individuals" and you might require more than this since your gut/body isn't really healthy yet. Additionally, the amount you need can vary and it isn't like there is some specific magic amount that applies to all people at all times and various states of health as well as your body's needs.

Personally I'd take as much as you can tolerate without diarrhea occurring. This is often done for Vitamin C dosing; the protocol is to start at a base amount and add more each day until diarrhea occurs, then to back off one level and maintain that dose.

Back to the Epsom salt baths. It has been alleged that the skin will only allow so much of it to be absorbed, and then naturally block any more coming in. While this may seem farfetched, the skin actually does this same thing in terms of making Vitamin D from the sun; After about 20 minutes, it senses it has enough and shuts down the process of making any more. It seems to make sense too because when taken internally the body does stop absorbing any more after it gets all it needs. So, perhaps the old Epsom salt bath is a preferred method to get magnesium and sulfur. I'd recommend giving the salt bath and/or footbath a try if it is practical for you; If you find it helps with aches, pains, and other things then stick with it.

A good absorption test would be if you have an ache or pain in particular joint that is accessible such as an ankle, knee, neck, wrist, or even hip. You can dissolve the salt in water and then soak a towel in it to use as a compress just on that area; If you get relief in 20 minutes then you know it is soaking in through the skin and also have a new remedy for injuries or chronic pain in joints–it is known that sulfur is very important for joints, cartilage, skin and blood vessels. Some people literally swear by Epsom salt baths and take them daily. By the way, the stuff is dirt-cheap and you can by a 10 lb bag of it for about $8.

In terms of food sources, you can get sulfur from both plant and animal sources. The plants have it in mostly a more direct form; The animals have it inside two sulfur containing amino acids: cysteine and methionine.

Best food sources for sulfur: the Allium vegetable family that includes onions, garlic, leeks, shallots, & chives; The cruciferous vegetables that include broccoli, cauliflower, cabbage, Brussels sprouts, radishes, watercress, kale, collard greens, and mustard greens; Also: asparagus, avocados, nuts, sweet potatoes, and tomatoes; Good animal sources include organic eggs, organic dairy, wild-caught fish, and grass-fed beef.

Notice the garlic listed and how we already mentioned it. Also notice some overlap with the previous list for magnesium. But also see how if you combine the lists that something should occur to you: If you eat a wide variety of vegetables and healthy animal products, then you get all of the important nutrients!

It is noteworthy that the sulfur comes originally from the soil. However, it can get depleted by heavy farming if it isn't replaced since the plants soak it up. Plants don't need too much sulfur to simply grow. So, modern farming practices use artificial fertilizers that are enriched in phosphates and very low in sulfur. They just want high yield and the fact that the crop is very low in the sulfur we need is of no consequence or consideration to them. Thus the organic farming and organic eggs/beef will have more of the important sulfur we are after because organic farmers must use natural fertilizers that have more sulfur in them. A grass-fed cow will eat more sulfur from the grass than a modern factory-farmed cow that is being fed the GE alfalfa and GE corn that just had the artificial fertilizers used to grow lots of it as cheaply as possible.

This raises another good point in favor or eating organic foods. And, this same thing applies to many more minerals and nutrients than just the sulfur; Many tests have been done that show organic foods have much higher levels of nutrients than GE crops or even non-organic crops that aren't GE. However, this can vary depending upon the specific farm, fertilizers used, and their specific practices.

Get plenty of sulfur: You can be sure to eat lots of garlic or take it in odorless supplements, eat sulfur-rich whole foods, and consider using Epsom salt orally or in baths. The Epsom salt has the added benefit that it is 50% magnesium, of which you also want plenty.

Let's move on to another one we added to the initial list: sodium bicarbonate. You probably have this in your home already, but may not be familiar with its name in Chemistry. We usually call it "baking soda". This stuff is flat out miraculous and going to be very helpful to you. I recall anytime we had stomach upset as kids that our mom would put a teaspoon in a glass of water and make us drink it.

If you research it on the internet you will find a very long list of ailments and conditions it treats; It is a true panacea. Of course it also has literally dozens of other great uses. Of course we put an open box in our refrigerators because it is known to kill mold, parasites, bacteria, fungi, and viruses. So yeah, it doesn't taste great, but it is well worth it to choke this stuff down pretty regularly. But how does it relate our guts and digestion issues?

Well, remember how your pancreas gets involved in digestion by excreting enzymes? Well your trusty ole pancreas turns out to be the place your body makes bicarbonate, which is what we use from the sodium bicarbonate or other ways we take in the raw material. Our pancreas produces and secretes the bicarbonate to neutralize acids coming from the stomach to provide the right environment for the pancreatic enzymes to be effective. In other words, it changes the PH level in the food sludge coming down so the enzymes don't get dissolved and destroyed by it–and so the small intestines don't either. This is part of why taking baking soda will alleviate acid indigestion, heartburn, acid reflux, upset stomach, and generally help out our digestive system. In fact, a single dose can make your stomach and gut feel and operate better for days.

Since bicarbonate is so important to digestion, it means that if and when we aren't getting enough of it then our whole digestive system goes out of whack; This includes not being able to fully digest proteins (including gliadin), and those then entering the blood stream.

Eating lots of sugar trashes your pancreas and impairs its ability to make bicarbonate, and so does eating acidic foods, drinking too much alcohol, eating spicy foods, and drinking sodas (which are very acidic). So, if you have been eating and/or drinking lots of these then your pancreas is probably struggling and sodium bicarbonate is really going to be a lot of help–in addition to cutting out the sugar, which you are already supposed to be doing on this program.

In addition to this, the pancreas produces your insulin, which you need to regulate your blood sugar levels and bind to glucose so cells can absorb it. Therefore, issues with the pancreas are directly related to diabetes; We know the graphs show correlation between glyphosate/GE crops and diabetes. Therefore, this either means people have also been chugging down too much high-fructose corn syrup and sugar along the same timeline, or that the glyphosate is also messing with our pancreas.

So, let's get some sodium bicarbonate in our bodies to help out this potentially damaged/struggling organ. It is important to drink it slowly, and a "teaspoon" is the type you use to measure in baking, not a spoon you stir your coffee with. Also, since you want stomach acid to help start breaking down foods, you don't want to take the baking soda right before or after a meal–unless you happen to be suffering from acid indigestion. One more thing that should be obvious: since it soaks up all sorts of nasty bugs and mold, you sure don't want to use the box from your fridge–buy a fresh box.

Take sodium bicarbonate (baking soda) orally at least 1 hour prior to a meal by dissolving 1 teaspoon in a tall glass of water. Sip that slowly over the course of 10 or more minutes. Do this two days in a row. Then take about 5 days off and repeat each week.

The next thing I added to our supplementing health/repair list is real/raw vitamin supplements. A vitamin is defined as an essential nutrient that you will get severely ill, diseased, or die without, which your body cannot make and therefore you must consume them in your diet. In general then, a vitamin comes from food. Since we are trying to help our body repair its self, we want to ensure we are getting all of these essential vitamins it needs in order to do so.

Of course nowadays we have vitamin supplements and/or multi-vitamins we can take to ensure we get enough of these critical nutrients if our diet isn't up to snuff. You might want to take them for the same reason. It is too long of a discussion to fully cover here, but there are differences in "vitamins" and I'll give you the quick lowdown.

Unfortunately, the pharmaceutical and chemical companies are the ones making 98% of these "vitamin" products. If you read the labels however you will see they aren't actually the same thing as vitamins. You will see they list the name of the vitamin, follow it by parentheses, and then list what they are putting in as a substitute like this: Thiamin (as thiamin HCl). These are technically known as "vitamin analogs" (meaning similar or the same as), or "pharmaceutical grade analogs" (PGA) to vitamins. While they tell us they are "close enough" or the same, I assure you they are not. Some may be a good substitute; Some of them have no benefit whatsoever and your body will not use them in place of a vitamin; Some of them are actually downright harmful to your health. In general they are a chemical witch's brew that shouldn't be trusted or used.

I have never seen "real vitamins" that weren't these FrankenPGAfakevitamins in a grocery store. You can't buy real vitamins there, so don't waste your time. Even health food store's shelves are lined with PGAs, and you will be hard-pressed to find 1 or 2 real vitamins on the shelves that are filled with hundreds. The reason for this is that the PGAs are made in bulk and the "vitamin companies" are just mixing them together and slapping a label on them; Of the more than 100 "vitamin" brands, 98% of them all contain PGAs made by just a few drug companies.

I'm a fan of taking supplements generally and also vitamin supplements. However, I only take (and only recommend taking), real, raw organic vitamins that are made from food. I strongly advise you to NOT take any PGA vitamins made in some drug company's lab. If you have vitamins already, look at the label on the back and if you see the list has parentheses and names in them, then throw that crap in the garbage!

Consider that neither Dr. Oz nor Dr. Sonjay Gupta take multivitamins–you think they might know something about them and not take them because they know they are mostly worthless or harmful pharmaceutical drugs and fakeFrankenPGAs? Seriously, you are better off not taking a multivitamin or other vitamin supplements than to take the fakeFrankenPGAs–seriously throw them out and do not take them! Either get real vitamins from eating food, or find the real vitamin supplements!

Naturally, in my book, "Total Health thru Complete Nutrition: Matt's Marvelous Shake" I reveal two wonderful vitamin companies and their products that are real vitamins and where to get them. You can spend hours trying to find the real vitamins like I had to do, or you can just buy my book–which has all the other information you need for complete nutrition and making that quick and easy shake too.

Consider using a real, raw organic vitamin supplement–particularly if you aren't paying enough attention to a healthy diet and eating a wide variety of whole foods. If you are a vegan or vegetarian you really need a good, real vitamin B12 supplement. Do not take fake pharmaceutical-grade analogs to vitamins; They are unhealthy drugs and don't work like real vitamins do.

The last thing I recommend supplementing is turmeric extract. This stuff is also healthy in multiple ways such as reducing blood pressure, preventing strokes, preventing dementia, supporting heart health, and more. The curcumin in it is what does the trick. It is the However, we are primarily interested in it because it is one of the most powerful anti-inflammatory herbs known. This will curb the inflammation your gut already has in response to all of the glyphosate and also its reaction to gliadin–in general you have basically had chronic inflammation. We want to eliminate that to support healing.

In addition to reducing inflammation in your gut, it will do the same in other organs and systems of your body that may have been upset by the glyphosate consumption and accumulation. One side benefit is it also deals with the type of inflammation that causes pain in joints, old injuries, arthritis, your back and muscles, etc. On top of this, it is known to be a big help to your liver in repairing itself–and we know the liver probably has taken a blow by dealing with a continuous consumption of the toxin/poison glyphosate. So, this is good stuff that will help your healing in multiple ways as well as improve your health overall. While turmeric is a common spice, you can't really get enough just adding it that way to foods. It will help some, but we are after a therapeutic dose. To get enough to do significant good you would have to eat about 1/4 pound of the stuff a day–that isn't going to happen. Luckily they make extracts that have that amount of curcumin concentrated into a single capsule!

Get a turmeric extract and take it daily as directed to reduce inflammation and to help repair your liver.

<u>**Summary and Review:**</u> That concludes our list of ways to supplement your health and healing during the program. The major part of it is eating plenty of healthy whole foods. You want to ensure you are eating enough protein and you can also use protein powder and/or Bragg's Amino Acids to supplement it. Besides the foods listed for good sources of magnesium and sulfur, using Epsom salt in a bath or orally can also supplement these. Garlic is highly recommended not only for the sulfur, but because it wipes out all sorts of bugs and nasty things, which will ensure your gut health isn't impacted by these. Beyond that, taking real/raw vitamin supplements, sodium bicarbonate, and turmeric extract round out all you will need.

During this time in the program you will also be continuing to take probiotics daily, using some black tea as a pre-biotic, and also ginger/lemon/honey tea for general digestive health and get rid of any nasty bugs and such. Strongly consider purchasing, "Total Health thru Complete Nutrition: Matt's Marvelous Shake" to support your overall health, ensure you get all of you nutrients each day, and to find out the best protein powder and real vitamins to use. Drinking "Matt's Miraculous Shake" daily will be a huge help in repairing and healing your gut, organs, and other systems in your body that were probably damaged by cumulative, long-term exposure to GE foods and glyphosate.

Chapter 16: At 1 Month

At this point you have now gotten off of both glyphosate and gluten to give your gut a break. You also gave your villi a break from corn, soy, wheat, and casein. To support its healing you have cleansed your gut, rebuilt your colony of gut flora, and focused on eating whole foods and doing some supplementing to provide the nutrients and minerals needed to feed that colony, make new cells, heal, and repair your gut physically.

The next step or phase of my program occurs after a month:

On day 30–or thereabouts–you now want to do a few things to continue this healing and repair process: Repeat the gut cleanse; Repeat the short fast; Take another round of high-dose probiotics for several days.

For the sake of completeness, after you do the above repeats, for the next month you are going to continue doing all of the things to support healing that you did after you broke your first fast. To help you do this, now would be a good time to re-read those chapters of this book to refresh your memory and it will also help you memorize and learn the contents better.

So, keep up with the teas, focus on whole foods, eat enough protein, and ensure you are getting lots of magnesium and sulfur via foods rich in those and Epsom salt. Stay with the baking soda regimen we covered, take your daily dose of probiotics and also the turmeric extract.

In addition to this, it is critical to stay vigilant about avoiding all sources of gluten/gliadin and glyphosate. Make note of any time you slip up or fall short. Did the holidays or some social gathering entice you to eat things you know better than to eat? Did you get weak or cave into eating a pizza or get sugar cravings so bad that you just said, "To heck with it, I'm going to eat it anyway?" Did you go out to eat with friends at some restaurant where you know glyphosate was on your plate? Did you just want fries or fast food so bad you threw your good sense and knowledge out the window? Well, it's time to renew your commitment and buck-up buttercup! We can't be perfect, and this program involves fundamental changes to diet and lifestyle. So just acknowledge where you may have slipped off the program and make up your mind to do better.

So, for the next two weeks you need to be focused and vigilant. You might want to really expand your purchase and use of whole foods during this time. Maybe you want to now learn some new recipes, meals, and cooking skills. If you didn't clean out your cupboards and refrigerator of the junk, this task is overdue; And for heaven's sake stop buying any more of it!

This is a very short "chapter" because you are just going to repeat the same things as the first part of the program and then do what you did for the first month. But I am making this chapter and the next one, separate chapters so they are easier to find and reference. If you are reading this as an Ebook, this is handy for navigation using the table of contents feature. The next step or change in the program happens at the 6-week point. But, be sure to read it now as it covers something important about the timing of the phases for you personally.

Chapter 17: At 6 Weeks

By this time your gut should be healed up physically. Also, with two rounds of high doses of probiotics and taking them daily, your colony of gut flora should be alive, well, and flourishing. This hopefully means your villi can now handle a bit of those things we have been avoiding.

However, I want to point out that each person's timing with this program will vary depending on three major things: how bad off your gut was to begin with; how much glyphosate you ate and over how much time; how well you stayed with the program and avoided glyphosate, gliadin, and did all of those things to support your healing and repairs. If you didn't follow the program very well, you might want to go another 2 weeks or more before moving onto this phase and the final one. If you are reading this now and haven't actually gotten to 6 weeks on the program, then you still have time to really be diligent with the program so you can progress through it more rapidly.

Okay, now let's cover this short phase. The things you haven't been eating to save your villi included corn, soy, wheat, casein, and eggs. The eggs only due to a possibility their protein gets a confused association or misidentification by your body. At this point we can start to eat some of these again.

However, this is something we want to take slowly; This is for very good reasons. Let's start with the casein. Remember this is the protein in milk and milk/dairy products like cheese. You've likely heard of people being lactose intolerant. Well, that is a form of sugar in milk. But there are also people intolerant or allergic to casein; In addition, we know it is fundamentally hard to digest. Since your body hasn't had any, let me assure you it might make some complaints and rumblings when you reintroduce it to your diet. A true personal story will help make the point.

I've never had any issues with milk, cheese, or dairy in my life—not one little bit. During college I took a humanitarian trip to a very small town in a poor developing nation. They only had one refrigerator in town and it was only used to keep sodas and beer cold–thank goodness for the cold beer because I was in a pretty hot jungle climate! At any rate, this meant they pretty much had no milk or dairy. There were a few dairy cows. But other than the people that owned them having fresh milk and cream, most people didn't get any; They certainly weren't making cheese or any other dairy products. I spent 5 weeks there. So, I had no milk, cheese, or dairy my entire stay. When I returned to the U.S. we flew into Houston International Airport. I clearly recall I had a huge craving for ice cream. While waiting for our next flight, I went to the food court and got a soft-serve ice cream cone. Man it was so good! Well, that is until about 15 minutes later when my stomach went into severe cramps. It was not at all a pleasant experience, and the aftermath wasn't pretty either.

I learned then, or developed a theory, that basically everyone is intolerant to milk and dairy. The main reason it doesn't bother us is that our body gets used to it and adapts to it. The body is known to do this in many areas. Even with milk it is known that if a child is allergic to it that you can give them just a little bit each day and slowly increase it to get rid of the allergy. It doesn't work in some severe cases, but it usually does. Since I knew I could fundamentally eat dairy, I just ate a very little bit at a time at first; I slowly increased the amount; In just a few weeks my body adjusted and adapted, and I had no further issues with it. In the next chapter we will also refer again to this technique working and why it does.

So just like my trip and 5 weeks off of dairy, you are now at week 6 and have been off of it. So you need to be cautious and re-introduce it slowly. Don't go chug down a glass of milk, or make a cheese fondue or you will regret it. If you drink coffee, you can start out with just a little 1/2 and 1/2 or cream. Maybe with cheese just a very small slice or two bites at a time/meal.

Corn may be quite similar to this. Some people are actually allergic to corn as well. It is also notoriously hard to digest–I won't mention the visual evidence of this the day after eating corn on the cob. Therefore, it is wise to also slowly reintroduce this as well.

Beyond this, imagine that if your gut had been mistaking these for gliadin, then you want to sort of give it a small test that it can pass. You want your gut to think, "Hey, I can digest these. This isn't gliadin after all. Okay, I'll no longer associate them or have something like a crossover allergy or intolerance of these." Now this would also apply to the eggs in terms of getting your body retrained to know they are clearly not related to gliadin.

Beginning at 6 weeks: slowly reintroduce some corn, milk/cheese/dairy, and eggs. Take them one at a time with a day or two devoted to very slowly reintroducing each in turn. After you are fine with the first one, you can keep eating it as you move onto the next. If you experience some complaints, just keep the amount small and stay with it. For the next 2 weeks, be sure to stay with the rest of the program.

Chapter 18: At 2 months: You are Healed!

Finally it is the time you have been waiting for and your program is basically complete. Your gut is healed and it is time to start eating gluten/gliadin again! It was important to wait two more weeks to accomplish two important things: ensure that your body doesn't confuse other proteins and gliadin; ensure your gut got fully healed.

Again I will remind you that if you didn't stick to the program well then you aren't ready to move on to this phase yet; Slackers and those lacking commitment and discipline need to now move to the back of the line, wait, and get with the program. Again, you aren't perfect, so don't beat yourself up about it and don't give up; Just renew your commitment and do better from now on. After you have been diligently on the program for 2 months then you can proceed with this step.

I'm sure you recall that you are supposed to be doing your gut cleanse every month indefinitely, right? Well, it is that time of the month again! Therefore, before moving on to the next part, here is what you need to do first, which is the same as at the end of the first month:

On day 60–or thereabouts–you now want to get ready for some gluten/gliadin and continue the monthly regimen: Repeat the gut cleanse; Repeat the short fast; Take another round of high-dose probiotics for several days. Then basically 4 days after your two months, you have a healed gut and a newly invigorated colony of flora that are both ready to start digesting some gliadin.

Similar to reintroducing the last foods at week 6, you need to take this very slowly and proceed with caution. The same reasons apply. Neither your gut, its flora, nor your pancreas have been forced to work on digesting gliadin, so they need to have very small doses and some time to adjust to doing it again. In fact, if you are like many people, you went "gluten free" long before you started this program. So, it is perhaps even tougher than it was with the corn and casein that you had only not been eating for 6 weeks.

Before we go any further, it is critically important to make one thing clear:

Even though you can now start eating gluten/gliadin again, you still cannot eat glyphosate. This means that in terms of things like bread that while you don't have to eat gluten free bread, you still need to eat only organic bread. The same applies to anything else with wheat or other gluten containing grains in it.

Similar to reintroducing corn and milk/cheese, what you need to do is start out with just a bite or two at a time for the first few days; By this I mean a total of two bites for an entire day. You can see how you tolerate it and very slowly increase the amount and frequency over the coming days.

Similarly to the dairy, this may cause a little ruckus and kickback as you begin to eat more substantial servings of it, or perhaps in the very beginning. However, as with my story of getting back on milk and dairy after my trip to the jungle–or the young child's allergy–if you keep eating it your body will adapt.

On the one hand, you now have a healed gut and healthy colony of gut flora so you should be able to digest it now. On the other hand, you haven't been using those embedded enzymes or your gut flora to digest it in a long time. It may take both of these some time to kick into gear, adapt, and your intestine may need to make more of the embedded enzymes as well. Consider that they are like athletes that have taken time off and gotten a bit out-of-shape and lazy. Putting them back into a workout regimen will work, but they need time to build up to any heavy lifting.

So, even if you have some side effects, don't think that means the program didn't work or that you should go back off gluten. In fact, it is best to stay with it and keep eating a little bit of it. Why and how might this be true?

Your body will adapt to most demands placed on it. It will also get lazy and not be able to deal with certain things if it has had time off from being forced to handle them and make what it needs to do it. Let me give a few brief examples. You can add these to my previous example of milk/lactose/casein and see that what I'm saying is true.

It is known that your body gets into shape in terms of growing muscles and also cardio as a result of stress. In other words, you must force it to do a bit more than it is comfortable with in order to basically signal it to get stronger and deal with what you are dishing out–or in our case what you are dishing in.

Your eyes make and secrete these chemicals called vasoconstrictors. When your eye's blood vessels get big, these come in and constrict them and "get the red out", which is the marketing slogan of Visine eye drops. Now if you start using Visine on a regular basis, your eye/body realizes it doesn't need to make these vasoconstrictors because it isn't being forced to deal with this situation. What happens is you become addicted to Visine and without it you will get red eyes that won't go away. The same happens with Chapstick/lip balms. Ever notice some people always have it with them and are constantly applying it? Well, normally our lips will secrete an oil to keep them moist, but once again if you start artificially taking care of the problem then your body gets lazy and stops making and secreting what it needs to handle the issues.

I had a friend I taught to mountain bike. Our first ride out she only made it up the first short hill and stopped. She doubled-over her handle bars and was gasping and wheezing. It was only then she told me she had asthma. Knowing what I do about the body adapting to demands and stresses placed upon it, I told her, "Well, that is an issue your body has with breathing. I recommend lots of heavy exercise and breathing. It will get over it." She seemed dubious about that and thought that it was unlikely her asthma would go away; She also said it would probably make it worse to keep mountain biking. With some encouragement she continued. Within a couple of months we were doing 30-mile rides and her asthma was completely gone. I saw her years later and she was still riding and still had no more asthma!

Now the only reason your body didn't somehow adapt to gluten/gliadin is because this wasn't due to a lack of demand or need in the first place, and because it was probably fundamentally damaged and prevented from doing so due to all the effects of glyphosate. In other words, you ingested a known toxin/poison over a long time so your body didn't even have a chance to be able to adapt and cope. However, now that you are off the poison and your gut and flora are healed, it is in the position to adapt and deal with it; It will buck-up and do whatever it needs to do.

Early on in this book I made the point about it being unwise to cover up symptoms, which are messengers informing you of a problem. This was part of why simply going "gluten free" was an unwise choice in my opinion. Now that the problem is known and has been handled, you can eat the gluten/gliadin again. Even if it takes some time for your body to adapt this is totally understandable and fine. It's fine because gluten wasn't ever the problem.

But, there is probably another important thing to consider: The longer you go "gluten free", the less capable your body will be in digesting it. As just discussed, lacking the demand/stress/need it will become lazy, out of shape, and not be prepared or making what it needs to handle gliadin. One example is that embedded enzyme in the cell walls themselves; Another might be that certain gut flora digest and feed on it, but if you aren't eating it then that strain may shrink in numbers, die off, or simply lose their own taste or ability to digest gliadin.

Summary and Review: At the end of two months repeat your cleanse, fast, and high dose of probiotics. After that, begin to very slowly reintroduce gluten/gliadin, but ensure it is organic so you aren't going back on the likely culprit of glyphosate. Your body responds and adapts to the stresses and demands you place upon it. Getting your gut and flora back on gliadin will force them to adapt and adjust; They will get in practice and good shape to digest it again.

This then concludes what is basically a 2-month program; The better you follow the program the faster and better your results will be. It may take more time for those that don't follow the entire program closely and with diligent commitment. If you are one of those, just extend the timeframes of the phases and redouble your efforts.

After you have concluded the program there are a few things to remember and continue doing: stay off the glyphosate; stay with the eating lots whole foods and getting your magnesium and sulfur, eat your folate and amino acids daily; keep taking probiotics daily; do a monthly gut cleanse; enjoy your life and improved health!

Chapter 20: Program Outline and Shopping List

As a quick reference tool and summary, here is a short outline of the various steps and timetable of the program:

Step 1: Stop eating all GMO/GE foods, ingredients, and sources of glyphosate; no sugar

Step 2: Cleanse and heal your gut

Day 1: Do a gut cleanse and fast the rest of the day; Drink plenty of liquids

Days 2-3 (4?): Fast, drink teas, use Bragg's Amino Acids, local/organic honey.

Day 3 or 4: Break fast slowly; Eliminate corn, casein/dairy, soy, sugar, and wheat/gluten

Days 4-5: Do high doses of probiotics and keep with black tea for pre-biotic

Step 3: Support healing, overall health and improve diet

Days 6-29: Focus on whole foods, amino acids, magnesium, sulfur, Espom salt, baking soda, and turmeric extract (possible raw organic vitamin supplements)

Day 30: Repeat gut cleanse

Days 31-32: Repeat Fast

Days 33-34: Repeat high doses of probiotics

Days 35-60: Continue supporting/supplementing with whole foods, magnesium, sulfur, etc.

Day 45: Slowly reintroduce corn, casein/dairy, and eggs

Day 60: Repeat gut cleanse

Day 61: Repeat high doses of probiotics

Days 62-63: Repeat fast

Step 4: Eat gluten again instead of avoiding and covering up symptoms and problem

Day 64: Slowly reintroduce organic gluten and wheat

Step 5: Stay clean; Eat healthy! After 60-day program: stay off glyphosate; stick with whole foods and supplements; keep up daily dose of probiotics; repeat gut cleanse and fasting monthly or at least every 2 months.

Shopping List

Here is a fairly complete list of things you need to help make your initial shopping easier for various program supplies and foods:

Fresh Lemon or Lemon Juice concentrate, Castor Oil, Psyllium Husk, Magnesium OXIDE, Milk Thistle, Azomite (or Brewer's Yeast); Black Tea, Ginger Tea and/or Fresh Ginger Root, Raw Organic Honey, Bragg's Amino Acids; Probiotics in capsules or Kefir Starter–multiple strains and high count of 20+ billion; Epsom Salt and/or Magnesium Sulfate supplement. In general shop for these: Fresh Veggies, Nuts/Seeds, Grains, Beans, Organic Meats, Fish, Dark Leafy Greens and Green Vegetables, Avocados, Bananas, and other foods from the lists for lots of magnesium and folate; Sunflower Oil, Coconut Oil, Real/pure Olive Oil; Organic Condiments like ketchup, mayonnaise, salad dressings, etc; Real/raw Multivitamins and B12; Fresh Garlic or Odorless Garlic capsules, Sodium Bicarbonate (Baking Soda), and Turmeric extract.

Chapter 21: Handling Relapses

I want to cover just two more things before we draw this book to a close and you begin reading "Total Health thru Complete Nutrition: Matt's Marvelous Shake". The first topic comes from my own personal experience.

My theory and program that I created definitely fixed my gluten sensitivity. I could do things like eat toast with breakfast, a sandwich for lunch, and pasta for dinner all in one day and not have any issues or side effects that I used to have.

However, I guess I'm human and after a while I got a bit sloppy, careless, lazy or unconcerned about the glyphosate. It seems problems get a lot of our attention when they cause discomfort and are active, but when the symptoms go away then we stop paying attention and doing what is best for ourselves. You might recall my story about doing physical therapy for my lower back problem when it was hurting, it getting better, and then I'd stop doing the therapy since it didn't hurt. So, this is exactly the type of thing that happened with glyphosate and me.

Just so you know what to look out for, here is a bit of what occurred for me. Sometimes I would be traveling and need food; I'd grab something at a questionable restaurant or even fast food (though I only eat at two of those ever that are likely the healthier ones). Holidays and family gatherings happened where I knew certain foods were a "no no", but I ate them anyway–and I must say I enjoyed eating them. Even after being off sugar for a long time, my sweet tooth got the better of me–it was about dang time for some ice cream and candy–sugar and high-fructose corn syrup be damned! My normal diligence, awareness, and label reading while shopping dulled and "no no" foods found their way into my home. One time I was out of bread and the store was out of the organic brand; Another time I settled for some GE bread at a tiny country store because I live so far up in the mountains. Suddenly, after not eating a doughnut in maybe a dozen years, I had an irresistible craving for those wonderful things just soaked in GE sugar and deep fried in GM oils! I must admit they were amazingly good and satisfying after all those years. These were those amazing cake doughnuts and I bought a dozen of them that must have weighed 3 lbs! I ate one a day–okay, sometimes two–until they were gone. They were so amazing I did that again about a month later.

Now you can imagine the consequence of all these behaviors and my basically having "fallen off the glyphosate wagon". I had a relapse and started having problems with my gut and gluten/gliadin again. I damaged myself. However, I was quick to notice it and took prompt action. I simply repeated my program and got off the poison again. I beefed up my probiotics, took a about a month off all gluten, and went back to eating healthy. After about a month I started eating some gliadin again a little at a time, but I was vigilant to ensure it was organic this time.

The point of this final chapter is to make you aware that this can happen. Maybe you will take this as a warning and avoid relapsing. If not, the point is to that you too might be human after all; you too might slip up or fall off the glyphosate wagon. You too might succumb to temptations even though you know they aren't good for you and will cause problems. And any of that is okay. If you fall off the wagon just stand up, dust off the glyphosate residue, climb back aboard and chug some probiotics, drive the wagon to town and fill it with good whole foods, cleanse your gut and you will be right as rain in no time.

I sincerely hope this book helps you fix your gluten sensitivity. A big part of it has to do with you following the program, and I know parts of it aren't easy and it requires a lot of change. But as I consider all of that, it seems to me they are all good and healthy changes that you really should make anyway. Additionally, I hope and believe it may also improve many other ailments, conditions, and health issues you and others might have; It will likely improve your overall health!

Please remember that "they" are against us knowing what is going on here and getting the word/truth out; So please spread the word about this book so it can help improve the quality of life and reduce suffering for family, friends, and others you know. Remember it will be a huge help to leave a review/testimonial on my bookseller's website detailing your success and any/all health improvements. Building up our own body of anecdotal evidence, informal case studies, and testimonials is probably the best way to fight back against the obvious attempts "they" make to refute the scientists, studies, articles, and evidence that are available and being done, but may never reach some mythical proof positive or be 100% conclusive.

I give my sincerest thanks to anyone who helps share the word and spread this book, and/or leaves a review/testimonial; To me this is about helping people and not about trying to get rich–after 3 years of writing full time, book sales won't even feed my cat. I just hope to change a few lives for the better and be of some help to others if I can.

Now the first of the two final things I want to cover has to do with diagnosing gluten sensitivity. You may recall that early on I said a good way to diagnose was actually a built-in part of my program; I also said that I think it is a much more accurate way than what is normally recommended. By now you should have the knowledge and understanding that makes this clear. The normal approach is to simply stop eating gluten for a week, see if the symptoms go away, and then eat it again and see if they come back. Based upon what you now know, take a moment to think about why that may be a flawed approach before reading onward.

Hopefully you thought about this: If the gut if currently and generally messed up and the gut flora are lacking, then you are only testing if they can handle digesting gluten/gliadin in that impaired state. You are not testing if you have some fundamental reason or condition that would be called "gluten sensitivity". In other words, it is more like testing if your gut is fundamentally healthy or not. What my program does is add in the whole process of healing the gut. After that you try gluten again and see what happens. If then the program works and you can eat gluten, then that means you aren't fundamentally or truly sensitive or intolerant of gluten; Instead it means that your gut was just so compromised and unhealthy that it was too much of a challenge due to gliadin being a hard thing to digest under normal circumstances; It may also mean that my theory is actually true: It wasn't really about the gluten, but instead "It's the glyphosate stupid!"

On the other hand, it is possible you could diligently go through the program and still not be able to handle gluten or gliadin. This might mean you have Celiacs and you definitely need to go to the doctor to have that checked out, tested, and address it. That situation could also be explained by a legitimate gluten sensitivity problem and thus you now have the correct diagnosis. There is also the chance that you had some other digestive issue or disorder that wasn't gluten related; It may have just flared up worse due to the tough gliadin. In that case, what happened is you weren't really gluten sensitive in the first place, but it turns out my program helped fix the other problem you did have–you misdiagnosed, but fixed the problem anyway.

All in all then I think going through this program will at least provide a much more accurate assessment and diagnosis. At best it will end up fixing your actual problem that the normal way to diagnose wouldn't have done, nor the advice to simply go gluten free, which would have covered up the symptoms and their important message to you. At the very best, all participants in the program may eventually show there really isn't such a thing as "gluten sensitivity" at all, but instead it is only a symptom and side effect of cumulative ingestion of a known poison over time that compromises multiple aspects of health and systems in our bodies–gluten/gliadin is then only the canary in the goal mine that is the first signal or warning of impending danger.

Acknowledgements and Closing

I wish to give my acknowledgments and express my profound gratitude to all those whom have researched, studied, written, and spoken out about the potential dangers of genetically engineered food, Roundup, Bt toxins, and glyphosate. I could not have learned so much and come up with my "working theory" about fixing gluten sensitivity without all your hard work and making your information available. I know that many of you have paid a heavy price of ridicule, attacks on your character and integrity, threats, lost jobs, and your careers have paid a heavy price for your good work and genuine concern for the health of humanity. So, thank you and please keep up the good fight.

There are "about the author" pages on my Internet reseller's websites if you are interesting in learning more about my background, education, and me. Beyond what is there, I do want to mention that in High School I studied Biology, Chemistry, and Human Anatomy and Physiology. In college I studied Human Health and Wellness, which included the fundamentals of nutrition and a healthy diet. Additionally, I have spent the past five years doing self-study on the Internet–including content from university courses–in Chemistry, Biochemistry, vitamins, nutrients, herbs, supplements, and many aspects of the human body and health topics. While I'm certainly no expert, I perhaps learned enough and researched enough to have some basis to figure a few things out. Beyond that, my personal experience and success story handling the gluten thing becomes the feather in my cap in place of other credentials; The proof is in the tasting of the pudding…non-GMO pudding that is.

May your gut be healed and your overall health improved!

- The End -

Also by this Author

You may be interested in my other published book. I will also be publishing about 4 more books in the next 6 months. Look for them and search my name at your favorite online book reseller:

Currently published: "Escape the Matrix and Explore Reality: A Guide to Radical Transformation and Empowerment."

To be published March, 2018: "Total Health thru Complete Nutrition: Matt's Marvelous Shake"

To be published March, 2018: "Harmonious Relationships thru Effective Communication: Resolving Issues by Healing and Dealing with Emotional Upsets"

Feel free to find and connect with me on Facebook (as Matt Stubbs or search for Rev.Matt.A.1 on Facebook)